Neurology Made Easy

Jon Adams

Copyright © 2024 Jonathan Adams

All rights reserved.

ISBN: 9798326301154

CONTENTS

1 The Neuronal Network Highways of the Mind ....Pg 6

2 The Brains Architects Glia ....Pg 17

3 Cerebral Symphony Orchestra of the Mind ....Pg 28

4 Electrical Storms Understanding Seizures ....Pg 37

5 The Plastic Brain Learning and Adaptation ....Pg 49

6 Language Unlocked The Linguistic Brain ....Pg 63

7 Sleeps Mysteries The Slumbering Brain ....Pg 72

8 Navigating the Maze Stroke and Recovery ....Pg 79

9 The Sensory Tapestry Interpreting the World ....Pg 89

INTRODUCTION

Welcome to 'Neurology Made Easy,' where the complex world of neurology unfolds in clear, understandable terms from A-Z. This book has been meticulously crafted for those who wish to grasp the depths of neurology without being specialists themselves. From the wonders of the human brain and its intricate functions to the challenges posed by neurological disorders, this guide is an attempt to demystify one of medicine's most fascinating fields.

Within these pages, you will find a treasure trove of information explained through deep analogies that breathe life into advanced concepts. Imagine understanding the brain's signaling system as easily as following a recipe, or grasping the delicate balance of neurotransmitters as if you were mixing the perfect cocktail. 'Neurology Made Easy' employs such vivid examples and relatable scenarios to make the subject matter accessible and engaging.

As we journey through the book, every chapter serves as a building block, piecing together the vast puzzle of human neurology. From the basic anatomy of the nervous system to the nuanced mechanisms behind common neurological conditions, we tackle each topic head-on with compelling, simplifying explanations. With a focus strictly on neurology, we'll delve into the medical aspects that govern nervous system functions and dysfunctions, leaving broader neuroscience concepts for another day.

By the end of 'Neurology Made Easy', readers will have gained a comprehensive understanding of the nervous system's essential roles, the importance of neurological health, and a newfound appreciation for the brain's resilience and adaptability. Whether you are a student seeking to clarify complex topics, a healthcare professional looking to refresh your knowledge, or merely a curious mind eager to explore the workings of the human brain, this book is your gateway to mastering the art of neurology with ease.

THE NEURONAL NETWORK HIGHWAYS OF THE MIND

The human brain's communication network is an intricate system composed of billions of neurons that act in harmony to control our thoughts, actions, and sensations. At the core of this system are the neurons, which serve as the messengers, transmitting electrical and chemical signals across a vast network of connections. The flow of these signals is critical for the brain to function, allowing us to respond to our environment, learn new information, and maintain the body's internal balance. Strategic points of contact between neurons, known as synapses, serve as relay stations where information is exchanged and modulated, making them pivotal in all neurological processes. This connectivity is what enables our conscious experience and underpins the operation of our body's systems, asserting profound influence on our behaviors, emotions, and health. It is through this comprehensive network that our brain performs its complex roles, shaping our every interaction with the world.

A neuron is the basic unit of the brain's communication network, functioning much like a specialized cell designed to carry messages. It has three main parts: the cell body, dendrites, and an axon. The cell body contains the neuron's nucleus with genetic material and typical cell machinery. Dendrites, branching off from the cell body, act like antennae picking up chemical messages from other neurons. The axon, a long, slender projection, extends from the cell body and carries electrical impulses away towards other neurons or muscles.

The neuron conveys information through electrical impulses called action potentials, generated by the sudden influx and outflow of ions across the neuron's membrane. This sequence of electrical charging is akin to flicking a switch to illuminate a room—it's a rapid, vital signal that travels the length of the axon. When an action potential reaches the end of the axon, it instigates the release of chemicals called neurotransmitters, which bridge the gap or synapse between neurons. Think of neurotransmitters like keys unlocking doors—they bind to specific receptors on the next neuron, influencing the likelihood of that neuron activating its own action potential.

A single neuron can connect with thousands of others, forming a massive, intricate network. The precision of this connectivity, and the delicate balance of neurotransmitters, is what determines everything from routine tasks like walking and talking to more complex brain functions like memory retrieval or the experience of emotions.

This framework of neuron structure and function is fundamental not only for understanding basic brain operations but also for grasping how medical conditions, such as Alzheimer's disease, impact cognitive and motor abilities. Medications designed to treat these conditions often aim to modulate neurotransmitter activity, illustrating how foundational understanding of neuron mechanics can inform real-world health solutions.

A neuron at rest maintains a negative electrical charge within its membrane, a state called the resting potential. This is due to a delicate balance of sodium (Na+) ions outside the neuron and potassium (K+) ions inside.

When a neuron becomes activated, usually by a signal from another neuron, the resting potential changes. This is initiated at the dendrites, which detect the incoming signal in the form of chemical neurotransmitters released by other neurons. If the signal is strong enough, it causes the cell body to generate an electrical signal called an action potential. The action potential is an all-or-nothing event; once the threshold is reached, the neuron will fire.

The action potential begins when sodium channels in the neuron's membrane open, allowing Na+ ions to rush in, which causes the membrane to depolarize, or lose its negative charge. Almost as quickly, these channels close and potassium channels open, allowing K+ ions to leave the neuron, repolarizing the membrane back to its resting state. This rapid change in electrical charge travels down the axon to the synaptic terminals.

At the synaptic terminals, the electrical signal triggers the release of neurotransmitters into the synapse, the gap between neurons. These neurotransmitters then bind to receptors on the next neuron, which can either start a new action potential or inhibit one from forming, depending on whether they are excitatory or inhibitory neurotransmitters.

Different types of neurotransmitters and their specific receptors play distinctive roles in neuronal communication. For example, glutamate generally acts as an excitatory neurotransmitter, while GABA typically serves as an inhibitory neurotransmitter. The balance between excitatory and inhibitory signals ensures that neurons can produce a coordinated response.

The entire process through which neurons communicate allows for the coordination of complex behaviors and cognitive functions, from simple reflexes to intricate decision-making processes. For instance, an imbalance in neurotransmitter levels is associated with neurological disorders, such as dopamine deficiency in Parkinson's disease. Treating such conditions often involves drugs that can increase or mimic neurotransmitters, thereby helping to restore proper neuronal communication.

This technical exploration of a neuron's communication process demonstrates the importance of each component as well as the dynamic nature of the nervous system. Understanding this can provide valuable insights into both normal brain function and the mechanisms behind neurologically based illnesses.

Consider the brain's nerve cells as the city's traffic, constantly on the move and directed by traffic signals. These neurons, like different vehicles, race along expressways—our brain's pathways—carrying vital information to various destinations. Just as a green traffic light prompts cars to go, a chemical signal in the brain tells a neuron to fire, sending its message down the line. Synapses, the junctions between neurons, act like intersections where decisions are made to stop or go. Neurotransmitters are the traffic officers at these junctions, guiding the signals to ensure they reach the correct route without a hitch. This intricate system of roads and signals in our brains ensures that from the simple act of tapping our feet to remembering a beloved melody, all run as smoothly as a well-coordinated transit system, making it possible for us to think, feel, and react to the world around us.

Here's a breakdown of how neurons chat with each other, like friends using different modes of communication to plan a meeting:

- **The structure of the neuron:**
  - **Cell body (Soma):**
    - Think of it as the main office where decisions are made.
    - Contains the nucleus, which is like the boss's desk with all the crucial

information (DNA).
- **Axon:**
  - Imagine it as a long corridor carrying messages from the cell body.
  - Messages (electrical impulses) travel down this path like a courier on a speedy delivery.
- **Dendrites:**
  - Picture these as the antennae on a television, receiving signals from other neurons.
  - They branch out around the cell body and catch incoming information, like a mailbox filled with letters from friends.

- **The process of action potential generation and propagation along the axon:**
  - **Resting State:**
    - The neuron is like a locked house when nobody's home, with a negative charge inside.
  - **Depolarization:**
    - A signal arrives, and the neuron 'opens the doors', allowing positive sodium ions to flood in.
  - **Repolarization:**
    - After the message is received, it 'closes the doors', and potassium ions exit, bringing back the negative charge.
  - **Propagation:**
    - This opening and closing of doors continues along the 'hallway' (axon), passing the message from the starting point to the end.

- **The role and function of neurotransmitters and receptors in synaptic transmission:**
  - **Neurotransmitters:**
    - They're the words of the message, each carrying different meanings (signals).
    - They're released into the synaptic gap (space between neurons) like throwing a paper airplane to your friend.
  - **Receptors:**
    - These are like your friend's hands, which catch the paper airplane and read the message.
    - When neurotransmitters bind to these receptors, they change the charge of the receiving neuron, starting a new action potential if the signal is strong enough.

- **How neuronal circuits integrate signals for complex behaviors:**

- **Signal Integration:**
  - Like a group chat, multiple signals come in and the neuron summarizes them into one 'decision' or response.
- **Learning and Memory:**
  - If a message route is used often, it gets a 'faster delivery', making it easier and quicker to send messages next time — this is how we form memories and get better at things through practice.

This simplified story paints a picture of the highly coordinated, complex world of neurons that allows us to function, learn, and enjoy life. It's like a busy city's communication hub that never sleeps, ensuring that everything runs as smoothly as your favorite coffee shop on a Monday morning.

Traverse the neuronal pathways in the brain as if you're following a meticulously drawn map. The journey of nerve impulses starts at one neuron, point A. Here, an electrical charge fires off when triggered by a sufficient stimulus, such as a sensory experience or another nerve impulse. The route then leads down the axon, a long fiber that acts as the roadway for the electrical signal. On this path, the impulse rapidly travels, passing through various gates known as ion channels. These channels open and close to let in and out charged particles that change the neuron's voltage, propelling the impulse forward.

As the impulse reaches the end of the axon at point B, it encounters the synapse, a tiny gap between neurons. Here, the impulse triggers the release of chemicals known as neurotransmitters. These chemicals cross the synapse and bind to receptor sites on the neighboring neuron, like a key fitting into a lock. This binding can either spark a new impulse in the neighboring neuron or stop one from firing, depending on the type of neurotransmitter released.

This journey, from initiating an electrical charge to passing the baton to another neuron, forms the foundation of all neural communication. Each step is crucial, from generating the electrical impulse to releasing neurotransmitters. This interconnected web of neurons creates a vast network, akin to a city's complex transit system, facilitating everything from the simplest reflex to the most complex thought. Understanding these pathways provides a window into the remarkable functions of the human brain and its ability to process, react, and adapt to countless signals at every moment.

Let's take a deeper look at the ion channels of a neuron, the tiny yet mighty heroes in the story of neural communication. Picture these ion channels as specialized doors in the walls of neurons that decide when certain molecules, the ions, can enter or exit, much like bouncers at an exclusive club.

First, we have the voltage-gated channels. They're like automatic doors that only open when they sense a specific electrical current. When the neuron gets excited and the electrical voltage changes, these channels snap open, allowing ions like sodium ($Na+$) to rush in, and start an electrical ripple down the neuron—what we call an action potential. After the party inside the neuron peaks, potassium ($K+$) channels open to let potassium out, calming things down, resetting the neuron for the next wave of messages.

Now, imagine ligand-gated channels as doors that require a special key—these keys are molecules called ligands, often neurotransmitters themselves. When the right key docks into the lock of the channel, the door swings open, and ions have the green light to go in or out, like friends entering with a VIP pass. This is vital for converting the chemical message back into an electrical one.

Mechanically-gated channels are more physical. Picture them as doors that only open when they're pushed or pulled by something - a mechanical force, like stretching. These channels are important in our senses, like feeling the wind on your skin because they respond directly to physical stimuli.

Now, prepare for a twist: neurotransmitters. They're the diverse crowd of molecules that work as messengers. Glutamate is like the life of the party, usually telling neurons to get excited, pushing them to fire off more messages. GABA, on the other hand, is the calming influencer who hushes the crowd, keeping things mellow. Dopamine and serotonin, they're the cool kids, associated with pleasure and mood, swinging the vibe of the neuron club this way or that, leading to complex behaviors and feelings.

Each neurotransmitter fits snugly into its own receptor, like a key fitting into a lock, triggering either a thumbs up or thumbs down for action potential. It's through this meticulous matching game that signals whip through the brain, enabling us to learn that new guitar riff or feel the rush of a roller coaster.

But if something goes awry—if the keys are cut wrong, or the doors get stuck—things can spiral out. Think disorders like depression, where serotonin might be off, or Parkinson's disease, with its dopamine dance going out of step. By unlocking these neural communication secrets, we could rejig treatments to get those doors opening and closing correctly once more.

So, there you have it, a brainy dance of doors, keys, and clubbers that let us experience life to the fullest. Understanding this elegant system puts us one step closer to helping when the neural network faces a beat drop.

Neurotransmitter interactions in the brain can be likened to a sophisticated party where guests communicate through a series of coded gestures and whispers. In this crowded room, each person has a special handshake or a wink that conveys a distinct message. These are your neurotransmitters, the brain's chemical messengers, each carrying a unique piece of information. When one guest extends a hand or raises an eyebrow, the recipient, like a neuron's receptor, knows exactly how to respond—maybe they smile and nod, or perhaps they step back, creating a lively dialogue of actions and reactions. This exchange is swift and specific; the messages have to be clear to cut through the noise. The effect of these interactions can ripple through the room, setting the tone just like neurotransmitters can excite or calm parts of the brain. Understanding this coded banter gives insight into how our brains process a multitude of signals to generate thoughts, emotions, and responses, always aiming to keep the party going smoothly.

Here's the breakdown on the stealthy yet crucial world of neurotransmitter communication, akin to a secret messaging system within your brain:

- **The synthesis and storage of neurotransmitters:**
    - Picture a small factory within the neuron, crafting neurotransmitters from simpler substances, then packing them into tiny storage units called vesicles – like loading texts into a phone before they are sent.

- **The release process of neurotransmitters:**
    - When an action potential zips down the axon to the nerve ending, it's like hitting 'send' on a message. This triggers the vesicles to merge with the presynaptic membrane and release their neurotransmitter cargo into the

synaptic gap, ready to shoot across to the next neuron.

- **The binding process of neurotransmitters:**
  - Each neurotransmitter searches for its matching receptor—like finding the right friend in a crowd to whom you want to whisper a secret. When they bind, the receptor activates or inhibits functions in the postsynaptic neuron, effectively deciding if the whispered message will be passed on or kept quiet.

- **The deactivation mechanisms for neurotransmitters:**
  - Once the message is delivered, it's not left floating around. The neurotransmitters are either pulled back into the original neuron, a process known as reuptake, or they are broken down by enzymes in the synaptic gap, much like shredding a secret note after it's been read.

- **The different effects of various neurotransmitters:**
  - Picture glutamate as the life of the party, making neurons more likely to fire and spread excitement. On the other hand, GABA is like a calming influence, making sure the excitement doesn't get out of hand. Their impact depends on which receptors they interact with, and it's the balance of these conversations that keeps the brain's activities smooth and coordinated.

Understanding these steps in neurotransmitter communication helps us grasp how our brains handle everything from reflexes to complex decisions. It's a buzzing world behind the quiet exterior of our skulls, with each handshake or whisper keeping the wheels of thought, movement, and emotion turning.

The myelin sheath is a critical component of many neurons, functioning much like insulation around electrical wiring. This sheath is a layer of fatty tissue encasing the long axons of neurons, which are responsible for transmitting electrical signals over distances within the nervous system. Myelin not only safeguards these axons but significantly boosts the speed and efficiency of electrical signal transmission. Without it, neural communication would be markedly slower; imagine trying to send a text message through a phone that operates on the earliest, sluggish cellular networks.

This efficiency is due to the way myelin sheath allows electrical impulses to 'jump' via a process called saltatory conduction, from one gap in the myelin layer to the next, rather like leaping across a series of stepping stones across a river, rather than walking the entire riverbank. The result is a much faster journey for the neural messages, ensuring rapid and precise communication across the body, crucial for everything from the reflexes that pull our hand from a hot surface to the complex processing needed to create and recall memories. Understanding how the myelin sheath operates helps us comprehend the sophisticated nature of our nervous system and why conditions that damage myelin, such as multiple sclerosis, can have such profound effects on bodily functions.

The myelin sheath is like the protective coating on electrical cables, but for neurons. It's crafted by special types of cells: oligodendrocytes in the central nervous system (which includes your brain and spinal cord) and Schwann cells in the peripheral nervous system (all the nerve pathways outside the brain and spinal cord). These cells wrap themselves tightly around the axons of neurons, forming multiple layers of membrane that create the myelin sheath.

Myelin's molecular structure is key to its role as an insulator. It's rich in lipids (fatty substances) and proteins, which together create a barrier that prevents electrical currents from leaking out of the axon. This structure is crucial because it means signals can zip along the neuron faster than in a non-myelinated neuron, ensuring rapid and efficient communication.

During development, as the nervous system matures, myelin production ramps up, forming sheaths around many neurons. This development can be influenced by a range of factors, including genetics, diet, and even experiences. Damage to these myelin sheaths can slow down or interrupt the signaling between neurons. That would be like having poor internet connection – messages don't get through as quickly or as clearly as they should.

One of the features that make myelinated axons so efficient is the nodes of Ranvier – small gaps in the myelin sheath. Think of them as relay stations along a long race track, allowing the electrical impulse to leap from node to node, a process known as saltatory conduction. These leaps greatly increase the speed of nerve impulses, like a sprinter jumping sections of the track to finish faster.

When the myelin is damaged, it can have significant consequences. For example, if myelin in the neurons controlling movement is compromised, it might result in muscle weakness or poor coordination. If the neurons associated with sensation lose their myelin, numbness or tingling can occur.

Multiple sclerosis is one such condition where myelin damage plays a central role, leading to a range of symptoms including movement and sensory disturbances. Current research into myelin repair, or remyelination, seeks to understand how to trigger the body's own repair mechanisms, or even use stem cells to produce new myelin sheaths. This could pave the way for restoring lost functions in individuals affected by such conditions.

In this chapter, we've navigated the brain's neural network, which operates like an intricate city grid, efficiently managing the flow of information much as traffic lights and signs direct cars along urban streets. Neurons function as the vehicles, transmitting signals rapidly across the neural highways. Myelin sheaths serve as insulation, much like the rubber around electrical wires, enabling high-speed travel of nerve impulses, vital for seamless communication. Synapses mirror busy intersections where neurotransmitters, acting as traffic signals, relay instructions leading to a complex coordination of movements, thoughts, and feelings. This elaborate system's seamless operation is paramount, as it underpins every aspect of human function, from the automatic reflexes to the richness of conscious thought. Understanding how this vast network directs the symphony of neural communication not only enhances our comprehension of the human brain but also has profound implications for addressing neurological disorders and injuries.

The human brain's networking demonstrates incredible efficiency and sophistication, comparable to the most advanced technologies and urban infrastructures. Through the delicate interplay of neurons and neurochemicals, akin to cars and traffic signals coordinating on bustling roadways, our nervous system performs with precision and speed. This neural network is at the core of every thought, decision, and sensation, allowing for the rich tapestry of human cognition and emotion. The complexities of our brain's functions underscore the marvel of neurology—how such intricate processes can happen within the confined space of our skulls. Reflecting on these analogies and explanations, we gain a deeper appreciation for the brain's role in our daily existence, and the groundbreaking scope of neuroscientific exploration. It's a testament to the wondrous capabilities embedded in every human being, fueling our continued quest for knowledge in the realm of neural sciences.

THE BRAINS ARCHITECTS GLIA

Settle in as we begin a journey into the brain's inner workings, focusing on glial cells: crucial components not often spoken about outside scientific circles. These cells are the supporting cast of the nervous system, much like a team of engineers that maintain the robustness of a city. Glial cells play essential roles, from providing scaffolding for neural pathways to insulating neuron 'wires' and even disposing of waste. They ensure that nerve impulses travel swiftly and efficiently, maintaining the health of neurons, and thus, the overall harmony of the brain. Their impact is profound, as they facilitate critical functions from motor control to cognitive processes. Today, we're uncovering these unsung heroes and their contribution to our understanding of neuroscience, an appreciation that is critical for anyone beginning to explore the vast landscape of the nervous system.

Glial cells are the brain's robust support system, each type with a specialized function essential to our neural well-being. Astrocytes, for example, are the versatile handymen, providing structural stability, nourishing neurons, and cleaning up excess neurotransmitters. They're like the support beams and janitorial staff in the skyscraper of our brain. Oligodendrocytes, on the other hand, wrap axons in a fatty myelin sheath, much like electricians insulating wires, which is vital for speeding up electrical impulses that zip through our nervous system. Microglia act as the immune sentinels, constantly patrolling and protecting neural pathways from damage and infection, similar to a city's vigilant health inspectors. Together, these glial cells maintain the brain's internal environment—its homeostasis—making sure that the delicate balance necessary for optimal brain function is preserved. Without these unsung heroes, our neural pathways would be like a city in disarray, with failed communications, collapsing structures, and unchecked threats. Their collective work not only sustains the mind's intricate operations but also provides a crucial foundation for advancing neurological research and medical breakthroughs.

Let's take a deeper look at the glial cells, the unsung heroes of the nervous system, and unravel their roles in a way that's as easy to follow as enjoying a cup of coffee with a friend.

Starting with astrocytes, picture them as the brain's multitasking caretakers. They are responsible for creating a balanced environment around neurons, much like a park ranger ensures that a forest ecosystem stays healthy. Astrocytes regulate the levels of ions and nutrients, essentially 'pruning' the space around neurons for optimal function. They also act as the brain's waste disposal service, mopping up excess neurotransmitters—chemicals used for brain cell communication—keeping the neural environment clean and orderly.

Now, imagine oligodendrocytes as electricians insulating wires. These cells wrap axons—the long, tail-like parts of neurons that carry electrical signals—with layers of myelin, a fatty substance that acts like the insulation around power cables. This myelin sheath is not continuous; it's segmented, leaving gaps known as nodes of Ranvier. Signals can 'jump' from node to node, vastly speeding up the electrical impulses that neurons send, enhancing rapid and efficient communication throughout the brain.

On to microglia, think of them as the brain's specialized emergency response team. They're always on the lookout for trouble—like pathogens or signs of injury—and when they find it, they spring into action. Microglia can change shape to 'eat' up invading microbes or dead cells and release substances that can either repair damage or, if overactivated, contribute to inflammation and potentially worsen the situation. They're like firefighters who are crucial to saving a building but can cause water damage in the process.

As we've journeyed through the roles of these key glial cells, we've seen how they contribute to the brain's health—maintaining a balanced neural environment, ensuring speedy communication, and defending against damage. Although they work mostly behind the scenes, their importance can't be overstated, much like the teams who manage the lighting, sound, and safety in a theater. It's the seamless operation of all these roles together that allows for the wondrous performances of the human brain in our everyday lives.

Consider your brain's communication system as the internet of an ultra-modern city, with neural signals as the high-speed data zooming through fiber-optic cables. Oligodendrocytes in the central nervous system and Schwann cells in the peripheral nervous system are akin to the dedicated technicians working behind the scenes. Their job is to insulate the axons, which are the equivalent of internet cables, with a fatty substance called myelin. Just as quality insulation on cables can drastically improve the speed and quality of your internet, this myelin sheath allows electrical signals to transmit rapidly and efficiently along the neural pathways. This natural engineering ensures that your brain's network can perform at its best, so every signal gets where it needs to go without a hitch—facilitating everything from your ability to click a mouse to recalling your favorite song.

Here is the breakdown on the incredible process of myelination, the neurological equivalent of wrapping your home's plumbing in thermal insulation to ensure optimal operation during winter:

- **Differentiation and Maturation:**
    - Glial cells begin as precursors, like apprentices in a craft. They mature through a series of steps, eventually specializing into oligodendrocytes in the central nervous system or Schwann cells in the peripheral nervous system, trained and ready to insulate neurons.

- **The Myelination Mechanism:**
    - Once mature, these cells start the myelination process, spiraling around the axons to insulate them. Think of them as workers wrapping layer upon layer of insulating tape around pipes. They use building blocks like proteins to provide structure and lipids to fill in space, creating a tightly packed, insulating sheath.

- **Nodes of Ranvier Formation:**
    - This sheath isn't continuous; it's dotted with unpadded gaps named nodes of Ranvier—mini stations along the axon. These gaps are crucial for the signal to 'hop' along the axon, allowing for quicker transmission, much as highway exit and entry ramps facilitate smooth and fast traffic movement.

- **Impact on Neural Signal Transmission:**
    - Myelinated axons carry signals significantly faster than their unmyelinated counterparts. Envision the action potential as an electrical surge that leaps from node to node down the axon, a process called saltatory conduction, delivering messages swiftly, like express mail versus regular post.

- **Maintenance and Demyelination:**

- The integrity of this insulation is vigilantly maintained. However, factors such as aging or autoimmune diseases like multiple sclerosis can wear down the myelin, resulting in slower signal transmission, much like worn insulation can cause plumbing to freeze and crack.

Understanding myelination and its analogies simplifies the appreciation of how our brain's communication lines are kept so efficiently. These insights not only enlighten us about normal brain function but also shed light on the critical nature of myelin-related diseases, guiding us toward potential therapeutic avenues.

Imagine the brain's microglia as the ever-vigilant security personnel of a large, bustling metropolis. Just as the city's first responders are always on alert, scanning the environment for any sign of trouble, microglia perpetually survey the brain for damaged cells or foreign invaders. Ready to leap into action at a moment's notice, these cells are the first line of defense, rushing to the site of potential harm. They clear away debris, much as emergency crews would clear a crash site, and can help initiate repair, similar to how a team would fix a pothole. They're indispensable, ensuring the brain remains a safe and well-functioning command center for the entire body. If there's a disruption—like an infection or injury—microglia are there, front and center, tackling the problem head-on to restore order. Understanding their role shows us just how dynamic and protective the brain's operations are, akin to a city that never sleeps, always working to safeguard its citizens.

Here is the breakdown on the dynamic functions and processes of microglia in the brain, presented like a well-orchestrated performance at a city's emergency operations center:

- **Detection Sensors:**
    - Microglia are equipped with a variety of receptors that act like radar systems, on the lookout for signals of injury or invasion. These can be thought of as the high-tech sensors and alarms employed by emergency services to detect problems swiftly and accurately.

- **Response Tactics:**
    - Upon detection, microglia can deploy an array of responses:
        - Releasing inflammatory molecules—think of these as the flares and barriers set up to control a scene and summon additional help.
        - Engulfing and digesting cellular debris and pathogens, paralleling a

clean-up crew that removes hazardous waste from an accident site to restore order.

- **Synaptic Pruning:**
- Like urban planners optimizing traffic flow by removing unnecessary roads, microglia refine the brain's circuitry by pruning synapses that are less active or weak, thus bolstering the efficiency of neural networks.

- **Activity Regulation:**
- The brain keeps microglial activity in check to prevent excessive responses that may harm healthy tissue. This is akin to the way a city's emergency coordinator ensures that response efforts are balanced and don't inadvertently contribute to the chaos.

- **Role in Neurological Diseases:**
- When microglial activities become unbalanced, they can contribute to neurological diseases—like overzealous first responders inadvertently causing additional issues. Recent studies delve into this aspect, exploring how microglial dysregulation plays a role in conditions like Alzheimer's and multiple sclerosis, and investigating potential interventions.

This approachable guide through microglia's capacities highlights the critical balance they maintain in our brains, ensuring it functions with precision and care. Understanding these details brings into focus the broader picture of our brain's health and our ongoing quest to safeguard it.

Astrocytes, with their star-like shape, are like the indispensable stage crew of a theater. They work behind the curtains, ensuring that the production—a seamless portrayal of your thoughts and movements—unfolds flawlessly. They regulate the environment around the neurons, like technicians controlling the lighting and sound, making sure each actor, or neuron, can perform their role perfectly. Astrocytes facilitate the delivery of nutrients to neurons and help remove waste, akin to the crew that sets the stage and keeps it clean. They aren't typically in the spotlight, but the show could not go on without them. These cells are key players in the brain's ability to operate smoothly, keeping the neural network humming along, ready for whatever scene comes next.

Here is the breakdown on the multifaceted roles of astrocytes, detailing how they're the brain's stagehands, ensuring every aspect of the performance is optimal from behind the scenes:

- **Support in Neuronal Metabolism:**
  - Astrocytes facilitate the transport of glucose from blood vessels to neurons, where it's vital for energy.
  - Break it down like caterers at an event, ensuring each guest — or neuron — gets the food — or glucose — they need to keep going.
  - They can convert glucose into lactate and supply it to neurons as an energy source, akin to a backup generator when the main power supply is not enough.

- **Blood-Brain Barrier Maintenance:**
  - Astrocytes envelop blood vessels in the brain, forming part of the blood-brain barrier that selectively admits substances into the brain tissue.
  - Picture them as the bouncers of an exclusive club, allowing only VIPs — essential nutrients and molecules — through the door, while keeping out potential troublemakers — harmful substances.

- **Regulation of Ions and Neurotransmitters:**
  - These cells help to balance the levels of ions and recycle neurotransmitters in and around the synapses, maintaining homeostasis for optimal neural signaling.
  - Think of astrocytes as air traffic controllers, ensuring that the skies — or synaptic spaces — are clear for takeoff and landing, so messages can be transmitted without delay.

- **Synaptic Formation and Plasticity:**
  - Astrocytes release factors that promote the formation of new synapses and strengthen existing ones, which is essential for learning and memory.
  - They're akin to trainers in a gym, providing just the right equipment and environment for muscles — or synapses — to grow stronger with each workout or learning experience.

- **Response to Brain Injury and Disease:**
  - Upon injury, astrocytes can multiply and form a scar to protect the surrounding neural tissue, similar to a construction crew quickly fixing a damaged building to prevent further collapse.

- In disease conditions, they can either offer support by cleaning debris and releasing protective factors or sometimes exacerbate the situation by forming tough, fibrous scars, complicating recovery efforts.

By covering these points with engaging and relatable analogies, we can transform the complexity of astrocytes' roles in the brain into clear, tangible stories. These star-shaped cells enable the smooth performance of the brain, much as the stage crew orchestrates a theater production from behind the scenes. Understanding their roles brings us closer to appreciating the delicate choreography that underlies our every thought and action.

Glial cells are the brain's architects, creating a sturdy framework for neurons, the cells responsible for transmitting information. These support cells not only provide a physical structure, like framing in a building, but they also assist in the brain's ability to adapt and change—a characteristic known as plasticity. This adaptability is critical for learning, as when you pick up a new language or musical instrument, your brain is rewiring and strengthening connections, much like updating an old building's wiring to support new technology. Glial cells also rally in response to injury, aiding in the cleanup and repair process, similar to a construction crew following a natural disaster. They play a part in forming new pathways, which can help the brain compensate for damaged areas, ensuring that essential functions can be recovered or preserved. Understanding how glial cells support brain plasticity opens a window into the remarkable ability of the brain to learn, grow, and heal throughout a person's life.

Let's take a deeper look at glial cells and how they're akin to a city's support system, from the electricians to the emergency repair crew:

- **Astrocytes Regulating the Neuronal Environment:**
    - These star-shaped glial cells maintain a balanced environment, regulating critical aspects like ion concentrations and neurotransmitter levels, similar to a building's maintenance system controlling climate and cleanliness to ensure comfort for its occupants.
    - They provide metabolic support by delivering glucose to neurons and then transforming it into lactate, akin to a power station supplying energy to the city's grid.

- **Oligodendrocytes and Schwann Cells Insulating Axons:**
    - Oligodendrocytes wrap multiple axons with myelin in the central

nervous system, while Schwann cells cover individual axons in the peripheral nervous system, much like insulation workers wrapping pipes to prevent energy loss.

- This myelin sheath is pivotal for fast signal conduction; you can think of it as high-speed internet cables that facilitate rapid learning and memory recall.

- **Microglia in Synaptic Pruning:**
- Microglia act as the urban planners of the brain, assessing and removing underperforming synapses – the connections between neurons – to optimize traffic flow, in this case, neural signals, which enhances the learning process.

- Following injury, microglia clear debris and can release factors that influence neuron recovery and plasticity, serving a role comparable to emergency services that both clean up after an incident and aid in the restoration of the area.

- **Glial Activation Post-Neuronal Damage:**
- After neuronal damage, glial cells receive distress signals, like a city's response team tuning into SOS beacons. They can foster a nurturing environment for neuron repair or, if overstimulated, contribute to scarring, similar to how construction efforts can lead to both the renovation and inadvertent obstruction of pathways.

By likening glial cells' varied roles to familiar services in urban management, we illuminate their indispensable role in supporting brain health, orchestrating learning and memory, and responding to injuries with a precision that maintains the brain's intricate functionality.

Imagine the communication among glial cells as akin to the hustle and bustle of a highly efficient office building. In this office, every department, like various types of glial cells, must exchange information rapidly and accurately to keep operations running smoothly. This is not unlike the way astrocytes, microglia, and other glial cells communicate using both chemical and electrical signals, ensuring that the brain's environment is perfectly calibrated for neurons to function. Just as memos and meetings keep a business humming along, these signals between glial cells coordinate defense against injuries, distribution of nutrients, and overall maintenance of brain health. It's this sophisticated network of communication that upholds the brain's intricate system, much as a well-oiled corporate machine drives a successful enterprise.

Here is the breakdown on the sophisticated communication methods of glial cells, relayed as if explaining the inner workings of a highly efficient corporate office:

- **Types of Signals:**
    - Glial cells use calcium waves to rapidly transmit information across long distances within the brain, much as an office uses email to share updates with the entire company.
    - They also release neurotransmitters and other signaling molecules for local communication between cells, paralleling a team using direct messaging for quick, targeted conversations.

- **Roles of Astrocytes:**
    - Astrocytes ensure that neurons 'talk' to each other properly by regulating neurotransmitter levels and cleaning up excess signals in the synaptic space, akin to a tech support team optimizing a network for better conference calls.
    - They influence the strength and creation of synaptic connections, much like a training department in an office facilitates the continuous improvement and learning of its staff.

- **Microglia as Threat Detectors:**
    - Microglia monitor the brain for signs of damage or invasion and react by engulfing debris or pathogens, similar to a security detail scanning surveillance feeds and neutralizing detected threats.
    - They can also send signals to other glial cells to recruit help, mirroring a security team coordinating with first responders in an emergency.

- **Oligodendrocytes in Myelination:**
    - Oligodendrocytes form myelin sheaths around axons, enhancing signal speed and integrity, much like technicians installing fiber-optic cables to upgrade an office's internet connection for faster data transfer.

- **Communication Dysregulation:**
    - Sometimes signals within the glial network go wrong, leading to diseases such as multiple sclerosis. This can be compared to

miscommunication in an office that results in project delays or system breakdowns.

- Disruptions in glial signaling can lead to neurons not receiving enough support or areas of the brain becoming inflamed, similar to how poor information flow can lead to bottlenecks and employee burnout.

By examining each point through the lens of common workplace scenarios, the complex and essential communication tactics of glial cells become as understandable as the daily operations of a well-managed office. This deeper insight into the cellular dialogue sheds light on how these unseen interactions within the brain are crucial to our well-being and cognition.

Glial cells in the brain function similarly to a city's sanitation department and defense forces combined. Imagine your brain as a bustling metropolis where neurons live like urban residents. Glial cells, specifically microglia, are like the city's waste management service, vigilantly cruising the streets to sweep up trash and dispose of it, ensuring the environment remains uncontaminated and conducive for the residents to function. At the same time, these cells are akin to the immune system's soldiers, patrolling for invaders like bacteria or viruses. Should a threat be detected, they act swiftly, like first responders to a crisis, engaging in cleanup operations, and signaling for reinforcements if needed. This dual role is essential; without it, the neural neighborhood could become cluttered and chaotic, disrupting the peace and functionality necessary for a healthy brain. By keeping the environment orderly and safe, glial cells allow neurons to perform their duties smoothly, contributing to everything from muscle movement to intricate thought processes.

Here is the breakdown on the crucial roles of microglia, the brain's own version of an emergency response and waste management team:

- **Types of Receptors:**
    - Microglia have various types of receptors that act as sensors to detect pathogens and cell damage.
    - Pattern recognition receptors (PRRs) spot common microbial features, not unlike a surveillance system recognizing the characteristics of common intruders.
    - Scavenger receptors bind to and engulf dead cell material, similar to a team trained to identify and remove harmful urban waste.

- **Process of Phagocytosis:**
  - Microglia engage in phagocytosis to encapsulate and break down waste or intruders.
  - They envelop debris like a sanitation team, wrapping up and removing garbage to keep the city — or the brain — clean and orderly.

- **Release of Cytokines and Chemokines:**
  - When harmful agents are detected, microglia release cytokines and chemokines.
  - These molecules act like urgent bulletins or calls to the broader health system, requesting backup to manage the threat to the brain's health.

- **Balance to Avoid Overactivation:**
  - Microglia must maintain a delicate balance to prevent damaging healthy tissue.
  - Think of it like a waste management team that must operate efficiently without interrupting the daily lives of city residents or disrupting other services.

- **Role in Neurological Diseases:**
  - When the functions of microglia malfunction or become overzealous, it can lead to diseases.
  - Similar to how an overwhelmed or faulty city service can lead to urban decay, overactive microglia can contribute to brain inflammation and disease progression.

Understanding microglia through the lens of city operations brings to light their indispensable role in maintaining a clean and secure environment for neurons, ensuring the brain's functionality and health are preserved.

Glial cells are indispensable to the brain's complex structure and function. As 'architects' and 'builders,' these cells provide support, protection, nutrition, and waste management for neurons, which are the primary communicators within the nervous system. Their actions are critical for the maintenance, repair, and plasticity of neural networks, affecting everything from our ability to learn and remember to our recovery from neurological damage. The healthy operation of glial cells is essential for our daily cognitive and physiological activities, underscoring their profound influence on our overall wellbeing. By acknowledging the pivotal roles glial cells play, we can better appreciate the nuanced intricacies of brain function and its impact on our lives.

CEREBRAL SYMPHONY ORCHESTRA OF THE MIND

In this cerebral symphony, each region of the brain emerges as a critical player, contributing to the harmonious execution of mental processes. From the frontal lobe's command of thought and action to the limbic system's regulation of emotions, every part synchronizes like the instruments in an ensemble, influencing actions, reactions, and interactions. This cooperative effort ensures the smooth performance of daily tasks and complex thinking, demonstrating the brain's profound impact on our overall functionality and experience of the world. In understanding the roles and significance of these regions, we gain insights into the essence and mechanics of human cognition.

Think of the frontal lobe as the assertive conductor of an orchestra, wielding the baton that directs executive functions—our daily decision-making, planning, and problem-solving. It's the decisive leader, ensuring that each section comes in at the right time, for the right duration, and with just the right emphasis. Now, consider the hippocampus as the principal violinist, leading the memory section. This vital region translates experiences into memories, setting the pace and tone for long-term retention, much like a concertmaster who ensures that the melodies linger long after the performance. Each area of the brain, then, plays its part in the concert of your cognitive experiences, working in harmony to enable everything from striking up a conversation to mastering a new skill.

Here is the breakdown of the integral roles and mechanisms of the frontal lobe and hippocampus, explained as if demystifying the roles of different members in an orchestra:

- **Frontal Lobe Integration:**
    - Coordinates inputs from various brain regions, similar to a conductor harmonizing the sounds of an orchestra.
    - Manages sensory information relating to sights, sounds, and touch, coordinating responses like a maestro leading the ensemble through a complex symphony.
    - Involves working memory to manage ongoing activities, much like a conductor keeping track of each musical score to direct the performance

seamlessly.

- **Hippocampus Cellular Structures:**
- Comprises neurons and synapses that work together to form and retrieve memories, akin to how the vibration of violin strings creates a resonant sound.
- Dentate gyrus helps encode memories, analogous to how a violinist's fingers adeptly press the strings to produce distinct notes.
- CA1 and CA3 regions of the hippocampus play a role in memory consolidation and spatial memory, resembling the violinist's bow drawing across the strings to sustain the melody over time.

- **Impact of Neuroplasticity:**
- Both regions exhibit neuroplasticity, which is the brain's ability to form new neural connections, similar to how a musician's consistent practice refines their performance.
- Like a musician learning a new piece, repetition in learning and experience can strengthen the synapses in these regions, enhancing cognitive abilities.

- **Cognitive Disorders from Malfunctions:**
- Disruptions in the normal functioning of the frontal lobe or hippocampus can lead to disorders, much like a performance afflicted by an out-of-sync conductor or violinist.
- Examples include the loss of impulse control likened to a conductor missing a beat, or memory issues paralleling a principal violinist playing the wrong notes.

Utilizing these analogies helps simplify the complex functionalities of the frontal lobe and hippocampus. It illustrates not only their individual roles but also their collaborative significance to the cognitive concert that plays out in our minds daily. By seeing these brain regions through the familiar lens of an orchestra, their mysterious operations become clearer and their importance in both health and disease resonates more vividly.

Functional connectivity is a term that describes how different areas of the brain link and communicate with each other. Imagine each brain region as a musician with a specific part to play. These musicians must follow the score, which represents the brain's wiring—its neural pathways. This interconnected network allows the regions to work together, coordinating their functions like an ensemble to produce smooth cognitive functions, the symphony of the mind. Just as musicians must precisely time their entries and match their rhythms to blend with the others, separate brain regions activate, sending and receiving messages at just the right moment to perform tasks ranging from recognizing a face to solving a math problem. This collaborative effort ensures that when we engage in any mental activity, the brain operates as a synchronized unit, much like an orchestra delivering a captivating rendition of a musical piece.

Let's take a deeper look at functional connectivity, focusing on the synapses, the brain's tiny junctions where 'musicians'—our neurons—exchange information. Much like players in an orchestra who share musical notes, neurons communicate through these synapses by sending each other complex messages. These messages can take the form of electrical impulses, the sharp staccato notes that travel at breathtaking speed, or chemical neurotransmitters, the prolonging legato lines that modulate the melody of our thoughts and feelings.

Diving further, the concept of long-term potentiation (LTP) is akin to a dedicated rehearsal process where the synaptic connections are strengthened over time. Just as a musician practices to perfect their part, repeated stimulation of a neuronal connection during learning makes that path more likely to fire in the future, solidifying the memory or skill being learned.

When there's a disruption in these connections, it's like a musician missing their entry, leading to an out-of-sync orchestra—the cognitive dissonance manifests as memory gaps, slow reaction times, or other cognitive impairments. Conversely, when all neurons send, receive, and synchronize their messages just right, the result is a harmonious mental performance, whether it's acing a test, navigating a complex social interaction, or adapting to a new challenge—the grand finale of our brain's daily concert.

By unpacking these concepts with familiar analogies, the intricate workings of the brain's communication system become less like an impenetrable score and more like a series of profound performances that are part of the vast cognitive repertoire each of us holds within.

Neurotransmission in the brain is like the silent nods and subtle signals exchanged between orchestra members during a performance. Imagine each neuron as a musician, ready with their instrument. The electrical impulse that travels down the neuron is the musician's preparation, the deep breath before the note is played. The release of neurotransmitters occurs as the note is struck, sending a chemical across the synapse, the tiny gap between the musician and the next, much like the space between violin bows and strings. This chemical message prompts the receiving neuron to continue the melody with an electrical impulse of its own. The whole process allows for a flawless symphony of cognitive activity, where every cue, every note, every rhythmic beat is passed along with impeccable timing, ensuring that our thoughts, emotions, and movements flow smoothly, much like an orchestra's seamless rendition captivating the audience.

Let's walk through the precise steps of neurotransmission, akin to a choreographed dance that's fundamental to how our brains function:

Step 1: Initiation
The dance begins in the sending neuron with an electrical signal called an action potential. It's like a dancer taking the first step on cue. This signal is a surge of electrical charge that sweeps through the neuron, caused by ions rushing in and out of the neuron's membrane.

Step 2: Transit
Next, the action potential travels down the neuron's long extension, called the axon, towards the end point known as the synaptic terminal. This is the journey down the dance floor, the dancer moving swiftly and gracefully to deliver the performance's crucial message.

Step 3: Transfer
Upon reaching the synaptic terminal, the action potential triggers small packages called vesicles, which contain neurotransmitters, to merge with the terminal edge. The neurotransmitters are then released into the gap between neurons, called the synaptic cleft. Much like a dancer leaping into the air to pass a prop to their partner, the neurotransmitters must make a leap from one neuron to the next.

Step 4: Reception
Across the synapse, these neurotransmitters are caught by specific structures on the receiving neuron, known as receptors. When the neurotransmitters bind to these receptors, they provoke changes in the recipient, like a partner responding to the movements of their counterpart. This can result in another action potential being generated in the receiving

neuron, continuing the dance of communication.

Step 5: Termination
Finally, the neurotransmitters must be cleared away to reset the synapse for the next signal. This is like the dancers finishing their move and getting ready to start again. The neurotransmitters may be reabsorbed back into the sending neuron in a process called reuptake, or they might be broken down by enzymes in the synaptic cleft.

In this elaborate dance, every step, every movement, is orchestrated to contribute to our ability to think, feel, and act. Understanding each movement provides deep insights into brain function and underscores the elegance of our neural choreography.

Neuroplasticity is the brain's incredible ability to change and adapt, much like updating the software on your phone to improve its performance. In more concrete terms, it means that the connections between neurons in the brain, known as neural pathways, can reorganize in response to new information, sensory experiences, development, damage, or other factors. For example, when you learn to play a new instrument, your brain physically changes to store the new knowledge. Neural pathways involved in coordinating movements and reading music strengthen with practice, while those not used as frequently may weaken. It's not just during learning; this process also comes into play when the brain recovers from injury. In this way, neuroplasticity is at work throughout your entire life, illustrating how dynamic and responsive your brain is to the experiences you encounter.

Let's take a deeper look at the intricate process of neuroplasticity, which is the brain's ability to rewire itself like a tech-savvy person enhancing their computer's performance:

- Synaptogenesis is the brain's version of adding new hardware, creating fresh connections to improve functionality. It's as if the brain is installing additional RAM to handle more complex tasks with ease.
  - Conversely, synaptic pruning is like decluttering a hard drive; the brain gets rid of connections that are no longer needed, streamlining its operations to focus on frequently used tasks, like a computer that runs faster after cleaning up unused files.

- When we learn something new, our brain releases specific chemicals, or

neurotransmitters, which help strengthen the synapses, akin to reinforcing the wiring in an electrical circuit for better current flow.
 - This process is similar to how, with repeated practice, a person becomes more adept at a skill—each action reinforces the 'pathway' through reinforced use, much like creating a shortcut on your desktop for quick access.

 - Neurogenesis, the growth of new neurons, is like upgrading the software version; it allows our brain to add new features and capabilities.
 - Even as adults, our brain can continue to create these new neurons, showcasing our brain's lifelong flexibility and potential for development, not unlike a smartphone gaining new features with each update.

 - The combination of these synaptic and neuronal changes has a profound impact on how we behave, learn, and recover. It means that after an injury, the brain can partly 'reprogram' itself to regain lost functions, a testament to its adaptability.
 - This is why someone who has suffered a stroke may relearn to walk or talk—because the brain can reroute functions to healthy areas, just like rerouting internet traffic to avoid a downed server.

Understanding neuroplasticity in this way illustrates just how dynamic our brain truly is. It's not set in stone but is more like a smart device that evolves, adapts, and improves over time, with our experiences serving as the 'updates' that keep it running optimally.

Consider the renowned chess grandmaster Magnus Carlsen and the neural ballet that unfolds in his brain during a critical match. His brain can be likened to a well-rehearsed ensemble, where each section - memory, strategy, foresight - works in concert to execute a flawless performance. The hippocampus recalls openings and defenses with the ease of a string section playing a familiar symphony, while the prefrontal cortex assesses the board and plots future moves, much like a percussion section maintaining the rhythm of the game. The interplay between different brain regions mirrors the coordination of an orchestra, each member contributing to the strategic dance, resulting in a beautiful melding of tactical execution and mental agility. Carlsen's cognitive abilities showcase how refined and practiced thought patterns, like those of a maestro leading an ensemble through a complex musical piece, can lead to mastery and brilliance.

Here is the breakdown on the various cognitive functions engaged during a game of chess, with each brain region playing a vital role in the match, much like musicians in an orchestra:

- **Hippocampus and Memory Retrieval:**
 - The hippocampus acts like the strings section, where memories of openings and game patterns are stored and retrieved with precision.
 - It is responsible for recalling previous matches, much like a violinist recalls the movement of a concerto played many times before.

- **Prefrontal Cortex in Strategy and Planning:**
 - The prefrontal cortex works as the percussion section, maintaining the beat—here, it's the beat of strategic thinking and foresight.
 - Functions include evaluating the current state of the game, anticipating the opponent's moves, and formulating long-term plans.

- **Involvement of Other Brain Regions:**
 - The parietal lobes contribute spatial awareness and planning, similar to a flutist following complex sheet music to play their part in a harmonic melody.
 - The amygdala manages emotional responses, ensuring the player remains composed under pressure, much like a soloist performing confidently before an audience.

- **Pattern Recognition:**
 - Just as a conductor spots themes across different musical pieces, the player's brain recognizes patterns on the chessboard.
 - This recognition leads to quick, efficient decision-making and can trigger instinctual moves based on familiar board configurations.

- **Role of Practice:**
 - Practice strengthens neural pathways, enhancing speed and accuracy of cognitive functions, akin to an orchestra growing more synchronized and expressive with each rehearsal.
 - As these pathways are repeatedly activated, they become more efficient, contributing to the player's growing expertise.

Understanding the parts played by these various cognitive functions elucidates how mastery in chess is not merely a testament to intelligence but an outcome of complex, well-tuned mental orchestration. With each game, just as with each performance, the mental orchestra refines its harmony, leading to the cognitive prowess exemplified by grandmasters.

Decision-making and creativity are like complex cognitive symphonies played out in the brain. Let's dissect these processes as if they were a music score. For a decision, the brain must first weigh options, which is the prefrontal cortex's territory. This executive part of the brain functions similar to the conductor, assessing the situation, anticipating outcomes, and making choices. At the same time, creativity taps into the brain's emotional core, the amygdala and the hippocampus, akin to woodwinds and strings adding depth and color to a musical piece. The amygdala injects emotional insight, while the hippocampus recalls past experiences to inform inventive combinations. Together, these regions harmonize, allowing complex thoughts to emerge seamlessly, much like an orchestra's blend of sounds culminates in an enthralling performance. These cognitive processes are foundational to our ability to navigate everyday life and respond with both logic and imagination.

In the intricate dance of decision-making and creativity, several brain regions play their unique parts. Let's examine these steps in cognitive processing in more practical terms.

The orbitofrontal cortex functions like a musician analyzing sheet music before playing a note. It weighs the pros and cons of actions, balancing risks and rewards to make calculated decisions. This region is critical in the evaluation process, assessing potential outcomes much like a musician interprets dots on a page to produce music.

Concurrently, the prefrontal cortex interacts with the limbic system, the emotional center of the brain, as they jointly orchestrate decision-making. This process can be likened to the way different instruments in an orchestra complement each other. As the strings swell and the percussion punctuates, the prefrontal cortex integrates logical thinking with the limbic system's emotional cues to inform choices, achieving a harmonious peak—a crescendo in both music and thought.

Creativity emerges from the hippocampus, where memories are stored like a library of musical scores. When the brain generates novel ideas, it's akin to a composer crafting a new piece by weaving together familiar melodies in unique ways. The hippocampus combines past experiences to generate new concepts or solutions, much like composing a new song from well-known tunes.

Finally, the reward system, which includes structures like the nucleus accumbens, plays a part in reinforcing creative endeavors. Similar to an audience's applause that drives a performer to continue, the positive feedback loop in the brain encourages the repetition of rewarding behaviors or thoughts, fostering further creative expression.

Understanding these steps clarifies not only how the brain makes decisions and invents but also the neural choreography that allows for the orchestra of the mind to play out the symphony of human cognition.

The brain, in its complexity and precision, mirrors an orchestra in perfect harmony. With each neuron and synapse playing its part, from the logic-driven decisions of the prefrontal cortex to the emotive rhythms of the limbic system, the brain conducts a symphony of thoughts, actions, and reactions that are central to the human experience. Understanding the brain's orchestral arrangement provides invaluable insight into how we function, showcasing the remarkable nature of its operations in all aspects of life. As we reflect on this marvel, we gain not only a better comprehension of cognitive processes but also an appreciation for the brain's ability to adapt and perform with incredible synchrony.

ELECTRICAL STORMS UNDERSTANDING SEIZURES

In the exploration of seizures, a condition characterized by sudden surges of electrical activity in the brain that can lead to a range of physical and cognitive phenomena. This chapter invites you to understand the fundamental nature of seizures, their causes, and their effects on the lives of those who experience them. Through a clear and straightforward narrative, we will explore how these episodes can disrupt the delicate balance of the neural network and the implications this disruption has for the individual. Whether you are new to the subject or seeking to expand your knowledge, this journey is about gaining insight into a critical aspect of brain function and empathizing with those who navigate this challenging condition.

A seizure is a burst of uncontrolled electrical activity between brain cells, or neurons, that temporarily interrupts normal brain function. Think of your brain as a network of electric circuits, with neurons passing signals to each other via electrical charges. A seizure happens when there's a sudden spike in this electric activity. It's like an electrical storm causing a power surge in the grid, which can lead to various unexpected and sometimes dramatic changes in behavior, movements, feelings, and levels of consciousness. If a person has repeated seizures, they might be diagnosed with epilepsy, which is one of the more well-known conditions associated with these electrical disturbances, but single seizures can have other causes, such as medications or high fevers. Understanding seizures is crucial because they're not just medical events; they also have significant implications for the safety and quality of life of those affected.

Normally, our brain's neurons communicate through controlled electrical impulses, each one like a messenger carrying information to coordinate everything from our thoughts to movements. During a seizure, this orderly communication is disrupted by a sudden, intense wave of electrical activity. It's as if these messengers are thrown into chaos, delivering their messages too quickly or all at once.

In a focal seizure, this wave starts in just one part of the brain. It's like an electrical fault sparking in a single neighborhood, potentially causing localized effects such as twitching or a brief lapse in awareness. On the other hand, generalized seizures are like a city-wide power outage, where the abnormal electrical activity rapidly spreads across the entire brain, often resulting in more widespread symptoms like convulsions or loss of consciousness.

The specific symptoms a person experiences during a seizure depend on where and how the electrical storm hits. For example, if the surge reaches areas controlling muscle movement, it may cause uncontrollable shaking; if it affects sensory regions, it might alter how things look, feel, or sound for the duration of the seizure.

After a seizure, there can be immediate effects like confusion or fatigue, similar to a neighborhood slowly recovering after a blackout. Long-term, recurring seizures might affect memory, mood, or other cognitive functions. Strategies to manage and treat seizures vary from medication to lifestyle changes, like stormproofing a house or a city to better withstand future electrical disturbances.

Understanding these processes gives us a clear picture of how seizures impact individuals and equips us with knowledge to effectively manage and respond to this electrical upheaval in the brain.

Seizures, like storms, come in various types and are triggered by different conditions. Imagine a focal seizure as a sudden downpour in one part of town—localized, possibly affecting just one limb or one side of the body, comparable to an isolated thunderstorm. In contrast, a generalized seizure is akin to a massive weather front that blankets the whole city, potentially bringing everyone to a halt; this is like when the entire brain is involved in a seizure, leading to a loss of consciousness or a full-body convulsion. Triggers can be as varied as the weather too; stress might set off a seizure like a cold front brings rain, while for some, flashing lights might trigger a seizure in the way that heat can spark a summer storm. Some seizures are like brief gusts of wind, passing quickly, while others are akin to prolonged storms, leaving a significant impact. Understanding these nuances helps us recognize seizures in their many forms and prepares us to provide appropriate support and response.

Here is the breakdown on the types of seizures and their triggers, crafted to make this complex topic relatable and clear:

- **Focal Seizures:**
  - **Simple Partial Seizures:**
    - **Motor Symptoms:** Like a glitch in a video game character's movements, these seizures may cause jerks or twitches in one part of the body.
    - **Sensory Symptoms:** Imagine sudden, unexpected sensations – a bell ringing or a light flickering – that only you perceive.
    - **Autonomic Symptoms:** These are like your body's background apps running haywire, affecting things like heart rate or flushing without your control.
    - **Psychic Symptoms:** They can be like a sudden wave of unprovoked fear or déjà vu, as if you've suddenly stepped into a scene from an old film.

  - **Complex Partial Seizures:**
    - **Impaired Awareness:** It's as if you're in a daydream, disconnected from the world around you.
    - **Automatisms:** These are repetitive, unintentional movements like drumming fingers or smacking lips, akin to tapping your foot to a song you didn't realize was playing.

- **Generalized Seizures:**
  - **Absence Seizures:**
    - **Brief Lapses in Consciousness:** These can be likened to the brief flickering of a light bulb, momentarily dimming without affecting the rest of the room.

  - **Tonic-Clonic Seizures:**
    - **Muscle Stiffening and Jerking:** Think of a sudden, intense dance routine that you can't control, one that takes over your entire body, first freezing it up and then moving it in spasms.

- **Seizure Triggers:**
  - **Environmental:**
    - **Flashing Lights:** Like a camera's flash interrupting your vision, these can momentarily "blind" the brain, leading to a seizure.
    - **Sleep Deprivation:** This is akin to driving on an empty tank, where your brain runs out of energy and might "stall," triggering a seizure.

- **Physiological:**
  - **Fever:** Elevated temperatures can make the brain's electrical systems overheat, similar to a car engine, potentially leading to a seizure.
  - **Substance Withdrawal/Metabolic Imbalances:** These are like suddenly changing the type of fuel in a running engine, which can cause it to sputter or stall.

- **Emotive:**
  - **Stress or Intense Emotion:** Much like a storm rattling a house, intense emotions can shake up the brain, sometimes triggering a seizure.

Each type of seizure and trigger corresponds to specific functions and reactions within the brain, affecting individuals in ways as varied as the weather affects a landscape. By understanding these connections, handling seizures becomes more intuitive, allowing for better support and care.

Seizure symptoms can be as varied as the unexpected things that can happen in a bustling city. Some seizures could cause muscle contractions, much like a group of flash mobs appearing here and there, suddenly causing a stir one moment and then dispersing. Others might lead to a loss of awareness, similar to wandering deep in thought through a busy street, unaware of the conversations and traffic passing by. There can be sensory disturbances, too, which would be like walking into a café and the smell of coffee overwhelming your senses, except it's a smell or sound that doesn't match the environment. And in some cases, seizures bring about abrupt emotional shifts—not unlike unexpectedly running into an old friend who brings a rush of joy, or an old rival who surges a wave of anxiety. By framing seizure symptoms in these everyday scenes, the strange and often sudden nature of seizures becomes less mysterious, grounding our understanding in the world we know.

Here is the breakdown on the specific symptoms associated with seizures, shown through a lens that brings clarity to their complex nature:

- **Muscle Contractions:**
  - **Types:**
    - Jerky Movements (Myoclonic): Comparable to sporadic hiccups interrupting speech.
    - Prolonged Stiffness (Tonic): As if the body is suddenly in an iron grip

of tension, unable to relax.
- **Neurological Basis:**
- Motor cortex disruptions provoke uncoordinated muscle actions, akin to signals getting crossed in a busy intersection.

- **Loss of Awareness:**
- **Manifestations:**
- Absence: Brief disconnections from the environment, like a flicker in a movie scene.
- Staring Spells: The fixed gaze, not unlike a pause button pressed during an intense dialogue.
- **Underlying Cause:**
- Wide network disturbances across the brain leading to pauses in consciousness, similar to a network outage affecting communication channels.

- **Sensory Disturbances:**
- **Variations:**
- Visual (hallucinations or loss of sight): Sudden changes in sight, as if the world is viewed through a distorted lens or a veil.
- Auditory (hearing loss or noises): Hearing sounds that aren't there, echoing the experience of having earphones producing sounds without being plugged in.
- **Brain Activity Disruption:**
- Malfunction in the sensory cortex can result in false perceptions, much like a radio catching frequencies that turn into static.

- **Emotional Changes:**
- **Emotional States:**
- Panic: An unexpected wave of fear with no apparent trigger, like an unexplained sense of dread in a familiar place.
- Ecstasy: A sudden, unprovoked euphoria, akin to an overwhelming rush of happiness from a surprise victory.
- **Limbic System Involvement:**
- Emotion-controlling regions responding erratically can lead to mood swings, similar to an audio equalizer abruptly sliding from one extreme to another without input.

Each symptom of a seizure reveals the intricate workings of our brain's electrical network and how small disturbances can have significant effects on our perceived reality. By understanding the roles and reactions of different brain areas during a seizure, we can better comprehend the experiences of those who live with this condition.

Diagnosing seizures starts with a thorough medical history, akin to an interview where the doctor gathers important background information. It's a step-by-step process where each detail helps to build a complete picture. First, they will ask about any factors that could have led to the seizure, such as recent injuries, illnesses, or medications taken—much like a detective piecing together clues from a crime scene.

The next step often involves an electroencephalogram (EEG), a test that tracks and records brain wave patterns. Imagine it as a seismograph for the brain, catching the tremors of electrical activity that may suggest a predisposition to seizures. Sometimes, an MRI or CT scan, which are like high-resolution cameras peering inside the brain, will be done to look for any structural anomalies that could be responsible.

Occasionally blood tests might be carried out to rule out other conditions, or to check for underlying metabolic or genetic issues — this can be compared to running diagnostics on a car to check for systemic problems.

Through this detailed process, the goal is to either confirm the diagnosis of seizures, determine the type, and identify any possible triggers or underlying causes, ultimately guiding the best course of treatment. It's a path marked with clear signposts, and following each one brings us closer to understanding the full scope of what someone experiencing seizures is going through.

Let's take a deeper look at the array of diagnostic tests used to unravel the mysteries of seizures.

- When it comes to an EEG, imagine it as listening to the symphony of the brain's electrical activity. During this test, doctors look at a screen that shows brain waves as lines tracing peaks and valleys, akin to the oscillations of sound on a music player. Certain patterns, like sharp spikes or slow waves, can indicate a brain prone to seizures, much as a trained ear can detect discord in a melody.

- MRI and CT scans allow doctors to look for telltale structures inside the brain, not unlike an architect surveying the integrity of a building. These scans can reveal areas of damage or irregularities, such as lesions or areas of scar tissue, which can serve as the source of seizure activity, disrupting the brain's normal electrical flow like a faulty circuit in a skyscraper's wiring.

- Blood tests serve as the body's diagnostics panel, checking for issues that might not be immediately visible but can affect its performance. These tests can uncover genetic markers or metabolic imbalances that could make a person more susceptible to seizures, much like a blood sugar test can indicate diabetes.

- A neurologist acts as the master puzzle-solver, taking all these individual pieces of data to build a comprehensive understanding of a patient's condition. By interpreting the test results collectively, the neurologist can identify not just the presence of seizures but potentially their root cause as well, setting the stage for effective management. It's a meticulous process of analysis where every result is a clue, every reading a step closer to the solution.

In taking this layered approach, each test contributes to a finely textured picture of neurological health, allowing individuals to navigate the complexities of seizure disorders with informed clarity.

Just as a city might work to quickly repair power lines and reset systems after a storm to restore order, so too does the treatment for seizures aim to return the brain's electrical activity to its normal rhythm. Some treatments, like anti-epileptic drugs, work like surge protectors, guarding against unexpected spikes in electrical activity that can lead to seizures. Other approaches, such as a ketogenic diet, might seem akin to switching to a backup generator—changing the brain's energy source to help prevent electrical outages. In more severe cases, surgery could be necessary to remove the damaged "wires" or "circuitry" that are causing issues, similar to how a city might replace an old, faulty power grid to ensure it runs smoothly. Each treatment method has its function, designed to stabilize the brain's delicate electrical network and prevent the disruption of a seizure, contributing to the overall resilience and wellbeing of those affected.

Here is the breakdown of the main seizure treatment options and how they work to regulate the brain's electrical activity:

- **Anti-Epileptic Drugs (AEDs):**
  - **Common Types:**
    - Sodium valproate: modulates nerve signaling and stabilizes electrical nerve activity.
    - Carbamazepine: works to dampen excessive electrical signals by blocking sodium channels in neurons.
    - Levetiracetam: binds to synaptic proteins and may modulate neurotransmitter release, preventing runaway electrical activity.
  - **Stabilizing Action:**
    - These medications act like finely tuned thermostats or circuit breakers in a home's electrical system, carefully controlling the flow of electricity to prevent surges that could trip the mains or cause a blackout.

- **Ketogenic Diet:**
  - **Metabolic Shift:**
    - The diet changes the body's primary energy source from carbohydrates to fats, which can be likened to changing a vehicle's fuel from petrol to diesel for greater efficiency under certain conditions.
  - **Neurological Benefits:**
    - May increase the availability of energy substrates that stabilize neuronal membrane potential.
    - Could reduce the excitability of neurons, similar to how better-insulated wiring reduces the risk of short circuits.

- **Surgical Interventions:**
  - **Types of Surgeries:**
    - Resection: like cutting out a section of damaged cable to prevent electrical misfires from spreading to the rest of the grid.
    - Neuromodulation (e.g., VNS or DBS): akin to installing a sophisticated pace maker that regularly sends signals to calibrate the brain's electrical activity.
  - **Goal of Procedures:**
    - Designed to remove the source of the seizures or to alter neuronal circuitry, much like overhauling an area of the power grid to ensure it can handle the city's electrical demand without faltering.

Each treatment is selected based on how it will help maintain the integrity of the brain's electrical system, ensuring stability in much the same way that a city's infrastructure is monitored and managed to withstand both everyday demands and extraordinary events. By exploring these methods, we shed light on the complex but ultimately manageable nature of seizure disorders.

Living with seizures often means making practical changes and emotional adjustments that can be as unique as the individual. This could mean setting a meticulous medication schedule, as regimented as a train timetable, to ensure that control over seizures is maintained throughout the day. Adjusting one's lifestyle might also involve creating a safety plan for 'just in case' moments, much like carrying an umbrella against unexpected rain. On the emotional front, individuals may need to navigate feelings of uncertainty or anxiety with the same care one would take when walking on uneven ground. Recognizing the triggers and learning coping mechanisms can be equated to mapping out a city, understanding where the potholes are, and the best routes to take. It requires open communication with friends and family, akin to sharing a roadmap of experiences, so everyone knows the journey ahead. It's not just about managing a medical condition; it's about reshaping a life to find balance and fulfillment amidst new challenges.

Let's take a deeper look at the day-to-day strategies that ground those living with seizures in stability and hope.

- Firstly, managing medication is like setting the hands of a clock with precision; it's crucial to take doses exactly on time to maintain therapeutic levels in the blood. Tools such as pill organizers, smartphone alerts, or even smart pill dispensers act as personal assistants, ensuring no dose is missed or delayed.

- For safety plans, imagine gearing up like a hiker preparing for unpredictable weather. This could involve making adjustments in the home to prevent injury during a seizure—padding sharp corners, or installing safety handles in bathrooms. Personal alert systems, similar to an SOS beacon, can inform a caregiver when a seizure occurs.

- Emotionally, techniques like mindfulness can be visualized as personal mental sanctuaries, offering respite from the whirlwind of emotions seizures can bring. Therapy acts as a guided path through a dense forest, helping individuals navigate their feelings with expert assistance. Support groups provide communal campfires, sharing warmth and stories that reassure and advise.

- Lifestyle adjustments can mirror the maintenance of a well-oiled machine, with sleep hygiene protocols ensuring restful nights like a scheduled downtime, and dietary regimens—potentially including a ketogenic diet—as specialized fuel blends designed for optimal performance.

- Identifying seizure triggers involves the meticulous collection of data, akin to a scientist in a lab, through diaries or journals, pinpointing patterns and catalysts to avoid potential seizure activity. It's detective work that can lead to more personalized and effective management.

- Finally, educating family and friends about seizures is akin to expanding a network of allies, strengthening understanding and emotional resilience. Informative talks might resemble pilot pre-flight briefings, where everyone is briefed on procedures before a turbulent journey, empowering them to act as co-pilots in care.

Together, these strategies form a multi-faceted approach to living with seizures. Every adjustment, every learned skill, fortifies the individual against the unpredictability of seizures, fostering a life of agency and community.

Danny Glover and Neil Young are notable figures who have managed to thrive despite their experiences with seizures. Glover was diagnosed with epilepsy at a young age and has spoken openly about the fear and anxiety that accompanied his seizures, which he refers to as 'brainstorms'. He has advocated for the importance of seeking support and not letting the condition define one's capabilities. His successful acting career, spanning decades, stands as a testament to his resilience.

Neil Young, the iconic musician, has dealt with epilepsy since his childhood. He has had to navigate the challenges of performing and creating music while managing this condition, a process that has required both adaptation and creativity. His story is one of endurance and determination, as he continues to inspire fans worldwide with his talent and tenacity.

Both Glover and Young have faced the challenges posed by seizures, but they have also demonstrated that through understanding one's condition, harnessing support, and finding adaptive strategies, it is possible to pursue and excel in one's passions and ambitions. Their journeys underscore the message that while living with seizures is an undeniable part of their stories, it is their accomplishments and influence that prevail.

Let's take a deeper look at how Danny Glover and Neil Young have carved paths through their careers while managing epilepsy, creating footprints for others to follow.

Danny Glover has fine-tuned his working environment to accommodate the unpredictable nature of his condition, much like a sailor might adapt a ship for stormy seas. Throughout his career, he has advocated for shorter working hours when necessary and informed directors and crews about his condition. This level of disclosure acted as a safety net, ensuring a rapid and informed response in case of a seizure onset during filming.

Simultaneously, Glover's outreach efforts can be likened to setting up lighthouses in uncharted waters. He raised the profile of epilepsy by speaking at events and working with organizations that focus on this condition. His honest and open discussions spurred a wave of awareness that not only educated the public but also sculpted a more compassionate narrative around epilepsy.

Neil Young's journey with epilepsy interlaces tightly with his creative process. Crafting music with the specter of seizures looming in the background, he learned to navigate this personal challenge, turning it into a source of creative fuel. Young's songwriting may well be a tapestry woven from the threads of his experiences with epilepsy, each lyric a stitch that binds the fabric of understanding a little tighter.

Both icons have taken firm steps to dismantle the misconceptions surrounding epilepsy. By sharing their stories, they've chiseled away at the stigma and carved out new ideals, contributing to a society that respects and empathizes with those who experience seizures. Their advocacy has resonated like a melody across communities, amplifying the importance of funding research and improving treatment options.

Their lives are powerful narratives, telling us that with the right accommodations, open dialogue, and determination, epilepsy can be a part of a successful and influential life. Through their advocacy and openness, Glover and Young have transformed a personal challenge into a chorus of support and hope for many.

Seizures represent a significant neurological condition that affects millions worldwide, requiring a comprehensive understanding to effectively support those impacted. The seizure experience, from the initial disruption of the brain's electrical system to the physical and cognitive effects, can profoundly affect an individual's life. Society's response, through medical advancements, supportive policies, and fostering inclusive communities, plays a crucial role in improving lives. As knowledge grows and awareness spreads, so does empathy, motivating a collective effort to ensure that people who experience seizures lead fulfilling, empowered lives. Recognizing the challenges and embracing the resilience required to manage seizures can inspire a more thoughtful and accommodating approach in every facet of societal interaction.

THE PLASTIC BRAIN LEARNING AND ADAPTATION

Neuroplasticity is the brain's remarkable ability to reorganize itself by forming new neural connections throughout life. This adaptability underpins our capacity to learn from experiences, recover from brain injury, and refine skills over time. It means that our brain's architecture is not fixed but is continuously shaped and reshaped by our actions and environment. This capability shows the brain's direct involvement in habit formation, skill acquisition, and memory retention. It is central to understanding how we become who we are—our personalities, talents, and even our limitations. Recognizing the power of neuroplasticity opens doors to potential treatments for neurological disorders and sheds light on optimizing our cognitive function. It is a subject that holds vast implications for personal development, education, and medical science, promising to guide us toward enhancing our brain health and unlocking human potential.

Neuroplasticity is essentially the brain's ability to rewire itself in response to learning and experience. For a clearer picture, think of the brain as a dynamic network, much like a complex railway system. Each station represents a neuron, and the tracks are the connections between them. Just as new routes can be established between stations to accommodate increased travel demand, the brain creates new pathways for nerve signals to travel in response to new information. This process allows us to acquire new skills; for instance, when practicing the piano, each keystroke strengthens the pathways until the melody flows effortlessly. Neuroplasticity doesn't just make learning possible; it also plays a critical role in recovery from brain injuries. When one pathway is damaged, the brain can often reroute functions to undamaged areas, adapting to continue functioning as efficiently as possible. This extraordinary flexibility of the brain underscores our ability to adapt, survive, and thrive in an ever-changing environment. It's not just a scientific curiosity; understanding neuroplasticity is key to unlocking treatments for brain disorders and enhancing cognitive abilities at any stage of life.

Let's take a deeper look at the complex yet captivating world of neuroplasticity through the lens of familiar, everyday visuals.

Synaptogenesis is like constructing new bridges between islands in an archipelago, each island being a neuron and each new bridge a synaptic connection. When we learn, our brain evaluates which 'islands' need to be connected to streamline the flow of information for a particular task or thought.

Long-term potentiation (LTP) is the process of strengthening these connections, much like a well-trodden path in a meadow that becomes easier to walk on over time. The more we use specific neural pathways, the better established they become; it's the brain's way of ensuring that important routes are kept clear and accessible for faster and more efficient use.

Neurotrophic factors are the brain's very own team of engineers. Just as construction crews repair and reinforce bridges to ensure they can handle traffic, these proteins repair and maintain neural connections, ensuring signal strength and neuron health.

Synaptic pruning is the brain's strategic management of resources, akin to a gardener trimming away the lesser-used branches to allow the more essential ones to flourish. It removes connections that are no longer needed, making the overall system of pathways more efficient, much like cutting redundant tracks from the rail network.

Lastly, changes in myelination of nerve fibers work like the upgrade from a country road to a superhighway. Myelin acts as an insulating layer around the nerve fibers, which increases the speed of signal transmission, making the delivery of information from one part of the brain to another as fast as the leap of electric sparks across the high-speed cables.

Through these processes, our brain continuously rewires and refines its functions, enhancing our ability to think, learn, and remember. It's a dynamic and ongoing system of renovation and optimization that keeps our cognitive abilities sharp and adaptable.

Imagine you move to a new town and find yourself driving to work for the first time. Your brain, with its neuroplastic abilities, is like the GPS in your car, initially offering several routes based on the traffic and speed limits.

As you repeatedly take the most efficient route, your brain, like the GPS, starts to favor this path, reinforcing it as the preferred one. This is how neuroplasticity manifests in learning—a repeated behavior strengthens neural pathways until they become the default for that action or thought.

In the realm of recovery, consider a person relearning to walk after an injury. Each step taken is like paving a cobblestone on a previously crumbled walkway. The first few stones might be laid down slowly and uncertainly. But as more stones are added over time—each representing practice and therapy—the walkway becomes firmer and more reliable. This is neuroplasticity at work during recovery, where the brain forms new connections to bypass damaged areas, gradually restoring movement through perseverance and repetition.

In everyday life, these neural adjustments are what allow a barista to memorize complex coffee orders or a musician to play a new piece from memory. The brain continually adapts, learning from each action we take, ensuring our skills and memories remain as agile as a stream carving its way through a forest, always finding the best path forward.

Here is the breakdown on the fascinating journey of neuroplasticity's role in learning and recovery, explored through clear analogies and palpable details:

- **Cellular Changes During Learning**:
    - Increase in Synaptic Efficiency: Much like enhancing Wi-Fi signal strength for faster internet speeds, synapses become more efficient at transmitting messages between neurons during learning.
    - Neurogenesis: Imagine a field where new flowers bloom; similarly, neurogenesis is the process of new neurons being born, providing fresh connections in the brain's neural network.

- **Molecular Events in Synaptic Strengthening**:
    - Role of Neurotransmitters: Glutamate is like the courier delivering messages; it binds to receptors at the synapse, strengthening the connection which is crucial for solidifying what we learn.
    - Changes in Receptor Density: Just as a busy store might add more cashiers to handle the customer rush, the brain increases receptor density at synapses to process information more effectively.

- **Formation of Neural Pathways**:
    - Synaptic Plasticity: Similar to laying down a new track for a train, synaptic plasticity involves creating and reinforcing pathways for efficient signal transmission.
    - Steps for Lasting Change: It's akin to building a house; laying the foundation (initial learning), putting up the walls (reinforcement), and finally, moving in (long-term memory formation).

- **Recovery After Brain Injury**:
    - Neurogenesis and Axonal Sprouting: In recovery, the brain can 'renovate' damaged areas, growing new neurons and creating new pathways like roadwork crews building detours around a roadblock.
    - Compensatory Changes: These are adaptative strategies, much like learning to write with your left hand if the right is injured, the brain finds new ways to carry out functions.

- **Synaptic Changes After Injury**:
    - Synaptic Plasticity: This is the brain's ability to adjust traffic flow across its network, redirecting it along new or rarely used paths to maintain function.
    - Re-establishment of Connections: Imagine a power grid that reroutes electricity after a power line failure; the brain re-establishes connections to regain and maintain its functions.

Through this narrative, we glimpse the elegance and complexity of our brain's ability to adapt, learning how our everyday actions lead to tangible changes in our most intricate organ. It highlights the potential for recovery and growth nestled in the microscopic details of our neural landscape, making the science of neuroplasticity as relatable as it is remarkable.

Synaptogenesis is the creation of new connections between neurons, which you can think of like adding new friends on a social network. Just as you form new relationships by reaching out to people, neurons extend their axons and dendrites to create synapses or contact points with other neurons. This is how the brain wires itself in response to learning or environmental changes.

Synaptic pruning, on the other hand, is more about maintaining a streamlined and efficient network. Imagine your closet at home; over time you get rid of clothes you no longer wear to make space and keep things organized. Similarly, the brain 'prunes' away synaptic connections that are no longer needed. It's a natural process that helps the brain stay tidy and functional by focusing resources on the most important and frequently used pathways.

Both processes are critical for a healthy, functioning brain: synaptogenesis adds necessary connections as we learn and grow, while synaptic pruning helps our brains eliminate redundancies and strengthen the connections that matter most. Together, they contribute to the brain's plasticity—its ability to change and adapt over time.

Synaptogenesis begins with neurons sprouting new projections like buds growing on the branches of a tree. Signaling molecules called growth factors act as nutritional 'sunlight', providing the necessary energy and directions for these projections to reach out towards each other. When an axon, like a vine seeking support, finds a compatible dendrite, they form a delicate connection much like two dancers holding hands for the first time.

This connection is made precise with the matching of neurotransmitter receptors, which function like unique keys fitting into specially designed locks, ensuring that every message sent across this juncture is received correctly. Over time, as the messages—or neural signals—continue to pass through, this synaptic bond is reinforced and consolidated. It is akin to the frequent exchange of letters between pen pals that strengthens a friendship, making it more resilient and intertwined within the social network of the brain.

On the other side of neuroplasticity is synaptic pruning—a meticulous spring cleaning of the brain. Neural pathways that are used less often are marked for pruning; it's like marking old clothes for donation, making room in your wardrobe for items you actually wear. Specialized cells in the brain, akin to waste management services, skillfully detach and break down these underused synapses.

The pieces left over from this process aren't discarded wastefully but are often repurposed. For example, a protein from an old synapse might be reused in the construction of a new one, much as a brick from a demolished building might be used to construct a new house. This selective trimming and recycling make for a brain that isn't cluttered with useless connections but is streamlined and efficient, each pathway like a direct flight route to its destination.

These processes illustrate the brain's dynamic nature—constantly building, remodeling, and refining itself. Through synaptogenesis and synaptic pruning, the brain adapts to our experiences, learning and recalibrating, ensuring we are prepared to face new challenges and absorb fresh information. It is the living proof of our brain's ceaseless endeavor to be more effective in its crucial role as the body's command center.

Just as a blacksmith hammers and folds metal to give it form and strength, our life experiences shape and fortify the brain's structure. When you learn a new language, it's like your brain is sorting through a tool chest, crafting new tools (neural pathways) for different linguistic tasks. And akin to a well-worn path made smoother by constant travel, familiar activities strengthen existing neural connections, making them more efficient. Each new experience you have is like adding a layer of paint to a canvas, gradually creating a masterpiece—this is your brain evolving, becoming more complex and capable with each stroke. Sometimes, certain areas of this canvas might be painted over or altered (synaptic pruning), streamlining the image, so the focal points stand out more vividly. These processes exemplify not just the adaptability of the brain but its incredible ability to refine itself to better meet the demands of our lives.

Let's take a deeper look at how our brains fine-tune themselves for peak performance through the intricate dance of creating and shedding connections:

When you encounter new experiences, your brain begins a construction project much like building a new bridge: it lays down fresh synapses to connect distant neurons, expanding your cerebral 'roadmap' and enabling novel routes of communication. Your first time learning a song on the guitar might be slow, but as neurons build synapses, you're essentially laying down the bridge's foundation over which your musical 'traffic' can flow smoothly.

With repetition, these newly formed synaptic connections are reinforced. It's as if the bridge is fortified with additional support to handle the increased traffic of neural signals, like reinforcing a well-traveled walkway into a sturdy pavement that can endure countless footsteps. The more you practice, the stronger and quicker the signal gets, allowing your fingers to find the guitar strings almost instinctively.

Synaptic pruning comes into play as the urban planner of the brain's landscape, identifying the less frequented routes—those synapses that aren't being used as much—and deciding they're not worth the maintenance. These are methodically pruned away, freeing up resources, much like a city might demolish rarely used overpasses to alleviate upkeep costs or make room for more essential infrastructure.

These changes—adding bridges and removing underused ones—significantly enhance our cognitive and physical adaptability. Just like a city updates its roads and transportation to suit the growing needs of its dwellers, our neural structures evolve to help us learn and execute increasingly complex tasks more efficiently.

Furthermore, when injuries occur, the brain's remarkable plasticity kicks in, resembling a city's detour system. If a main pathway is damaged, alternate routes are established to retain function. This ability of the brain to reroute and rebuild itself manifests in the rehabilitation from physical injuries and the resilience seen in overcoming cognitive obstacles.

Understanding these processes sheds light on the extraordinary adaptability of the human brain, revealing a world of neural architecture that is constantly being sculpted—carefully wired and pruned—by our everyday experiences and actions.

Consider forming and retaining memories to be like walking a path through a dense forest. The first time you venture through, you might struggle to find your way, pushing aside branches and stepping over roots. As you travel the same path repeatedly, though, your footsteps begin to clear the underbrush. A well-defined trail takes shape, making it easier to follow the route without thinking too much about it. Similarly, when you first learn a fact or have a new experience, your brain begins the process of forming a memory. This path is the neural connection through which signals travel. Each time you recall this information, you're reinforcing this pathway, making it more prominent and accessible in the brain's complex network. Just like a well-trodden trail that's simple to walk, a frequently recalled memory becomes easier to retrieve, until it is stored firmly and can be accessed without effort. This analogy shows the practical, continual process of how our actions—our repeated recollections—embed memories deep within our mind's expansive landscape.

Here is the breakdown on the intricate process of memory formation and retrieval in our brains, outlined with analogies to make each component tangible:

- **Initial Encoding of Information**
  - This is like taking a mental photograph of an event or fact, capturing the essence of the experience in your mind.
  - Sensory information is processed by the relevant sensory areas of the cortex - the 'camera lens' through which the brain focuses on details.

- **Process of Consolidation**
  - The brain acts as a meticulous librarian, cataloging these photographic memories and storing them neatly on the 'bookshelves' of the mind.
  - During sleep, the hippocampus 'reviews' and 'files' away these experiences for long-term storage - it's like the brain's after-hours sorting session to ensure everything is in order for future reference.

- **Role of the Hippocampus**
  - The hippocampus is akin to a central processing unit, crucial for transforming fresh experiences into storable memory data.
  - It associates different aspects of a memory, such as sights and smells, linking them together like a network of interconnected roads on a map leading to the same landmark.

- **Memory Retrieval**
  - Retrieving a memory is like selecting a book from a shelf; the more frequently you access it, the more prominently it's placed, and the easier it is to find.
  - Environmental cues or emotional states can prompt memory retrieval, functioning as 'reminders' or 'hints' that guide you to the correct 'book' amongst many.

- **Memory Distortion Over Time**
  - With each recall, memories can change subtly, paralleling how a story

can evolve each time it's retold.

- Like in a game of telephone, the original message may get altered as it passes through various 'neural players,' affected by new experiences or interpretations.

As you move through life, recall and reflect on these memories, your brain adjusts this internal library. Connections are strengthened, information is cross-referenced, and occasionally, details are reshaped. Understanding this process highlights both the durability and the delicate nature of how we remember, emphasizing the ever-changing landscape of our cognitive experiences.

The stories of Gabby Giffords and Pat Martino are profound illustrations of the brain's capacity to heal and reconfigure itself through neuroplasticity. Giffords, a former U.S. congresswoman, suffered a severe brain injury from a gunshot wound that left her with significant speech and movement impairments. Through an intensive rehabilitation process, where she relearned to speak and walk, Giffords used the fundamental principles of repetition and practice to gradually rebuild her neural pathways. The persistence paid off — today, she speaks and moves with a level of fluidity that once seemed unattainable, showcasing the potential for recovery post-injury.

Renowned jazz guitarist Pat Martino offers another extraordinary example. After contracting an aneurysm, he lost nearly all of his memory, including his ability to play the guitar. Despite this overwhelming setback, Martino re-taught himself the guitar from scratch, leveraging the inherent plasticity of his brain to form new memory circuits and skills. His return to performing at an elite level is not just a testament to his determination but also to the adaptability of the human brain.

Both Giffords and Martino exemplify the concept of neuroplasticity — the brain's remarkable ability to adapt and refine its structure and function in response to experiences. Their journeys provide real-world context to the theory, validating the brain's malleable nature and the impressive potential that lies within focused and consistent rehabilitation efforts.

Let's take a deeper look at the incredible paths Giffords and Martino took, navigating through the complexities of brain recovery to regain and re-master their lives' passions.

Gabby Giffords, after her injury, embarked on a tailored neurorehabilitation regimen designed to rekindle the brain's communication routes. Her therapy likely included speech-language therapy to help rebuild her language skills—a process not unlike re-learning how to compose a symphony of words. Additionally, physical therapy aimed at her motor skills served to reawaken her brain's ability to coordinate body movements, as if she were teaching her limbs to dance again. These consistent activities provided the 'exercise' her brain needed to forge new neural pathways, circumventing the damages to restore her speech and mobility.

As for Pat Martino, imagine his reintroduction to the guitar as someone rediscovering their own hometown after many years. He would start with the guitar itself, touching and plucking each string, leading to basic chords and eventually re-learning complex compositions. Each step reinforced his finger dexterity and reinvigorated the musical areas of his brain, akin to a forgotten language resurfacing word by word. His auditory cortex tuned in to the sound of each note, and his motor cortex synchronized the intricate finger movements required for those notes to resonate.

Both journeys utilized the plastic nature of the brain in their recovery. Synaptic plasticity, where existing connections strengthen, and cortical plasticity, involving changes in the brain's structure, were likely integral. Critical to this was the production of neurotrophic factors—proteins that serve as the brain's version of fertilizers, nourishing neurons to support and encourage growth.

Through deduced analogies, we see that their targeted therapies engaged both the physical and cognitive faculties, essentially re-mapping their brains to regain function. It stands as a testament to the resilience not only of Giffords and Martino but of the human brain's inherent potential for healing and adaptation.

While the brain's neuroplastic capabilities are a powerful testament to our potential for change, it's important to acknowledge that various factors can influence this plasticity. Age is one such factor; in general, younger brains tend to be more malleable and quicker to adapt. Think of a child learning a new language with apparent ease compared to an adult, for whom the process is often more arduous. As we age, some of the brain's capacity for forming new connections does slow down, but it never loses this ability entirely—it just may take more effort and time.

The severity of neurological damage is another critical factor. The more extensive the injury, the more challenging it may be for the brain to reestablish lost connections. Consider a heavily trafficked bridge that collapses; the disruption is far greater and requires more complex engineering to repair compared to a small footbridge. However, with targeted rehabilitation and therapy, even brains with significant injuries can find new pathways and methods of functioning. It's important to recognize that each individual's journey with neuroplasticity is unique, influenced by their specific circumstances and the inherent resilience of their neural networks.

Following a brain injury, the body initiates a process akin to a city's emergency response after a disaster—there's a rush to assess damage, clear debris, and lay plans for repair. The brain's immediate reaction involves neural shock, where damaged areas cease their usual activities. Inflammation swiftly follows as the brain's clean-up crew, targeting and clearing cellular debris. After this, akin to fixing roads and buildings, the brain begins the longer process of rewiring and rehabilitation.

During recovery, age plays a crucial role akin to the difference in speed and ease with which young saplings versus old trees can take root and flourish after a forest fire. Younger brains tend to show a quicker restoration of nervous pathways, much like how quickly new plants sprout up. In contrast, older individuals may require more targeted stimulation to foster regrowth. Techniques such as mental exercises that challenge memory, problem-solving and motor skills training, can act like greenhouses, cultivating the conditions needed for brain recovery.

Therapeutic strategies for rehabilitation might involve physical therapy, teaching the body to reclaim movements and strength much like reconstructing a building from its remaining structure. Occupational therapy helps individuals relearn daily tasks, steadily reestablishing the routine networks akin to restarting a city's public services. Cognitive therapies work on the principles of repetition and challenge, reinforcing neural pathways through continued use, much like repaving a road to handle traffic smoothly.

Moreover, neuromodulation techniques, including transcranial magnetic stimulation (TMS) and deep brain stimulation (DBS), are like the introduction of advanced technology in rebuilding efforts, providing targeted, high-tech assistance to the recovery process. Additionally, neuropharmacological agents that promote brain growth or synaptic strength can offer chemical support, akin to providing nutritional supplements to support the body's healing.

Overall, understanding each facet of neuroplastic recovery provides a holistic view of the journey from injury toward healing, recognizing the brain's intricate yet resilient nature in adapting to new challenges. This understanding offers not just insight but also hope for those undergoing recovery, that with time and appropriate therapy, improvement and adaptation are within reach.

To cultivate a garden of the mind that's as fertile as Earth's richest soils, consider incorporating a blend of mental exercises and physical activities into your daily routine. Mental exercises are like planting seeds of knowledge and skill in your brain; each new mathematical problem you tackle or each foreign word you memorize nurtures these seeds, which can sprout into robust pathways of understanding. Crossword puzzles, learning a new language, or even musical training are akin to giving these seeds the right amount of sunlight—they challenge your brain to adapt and grow.

Physical activity, on the other hand, waters and fertilizes this cerebral garden. Aerobic exercises such as running, swimming, or even brisk walking increase the flow of blood and oxygen to your brain, much like nourishing rain encourages a recently sown field to flourish. This not only supports the maintenance of existing neural connections but also encourages the growth of new ones. By balancing cognitive challenges with physical health, you foster an optimal environment for neuroplasticity, ensuring that your brain's landscape is rich with connections, primed for learning, and resilient against aging.

Here is the breakdown on the intricate ways in which mental exercises and physical activity can synergistically bolster brain health:

- **Mental Exercises:**
  - **Cognitive Activities:**
    - Puzzles like crosswords or Sudoku predominantly engage the prefrontal cortex, our brain's problem-solving command center.
    - Learning a new language activates the temporal lobes, which are

involved in processing auditory information and are crucial for memory.
- Playing musical instruments stimulates a broad network of brain regions, including those responsible for coordination, auditory processing, and creative thinking.

- **Synaptic Plasticity:**
- These activities encourage the brain to form new synapses, akin to paving new pathways in a dense forest for more efficient travel.
- They also strengthen existing neural networks, making the transmission of electrical signals as smooth as an upgraded high-speed internet connection.

- **Physical Activities:**
  - **Exercises and Brain Blood Flow:**
- Aerobic exercises, such as running or swimming, enhance cerebral blood flow, showering the brain's garden with the necessary nutrients and oxygen, much like a refreshing rain.
- These physical activities also promote synaptogenesis, where the brain grows new synaptic connections, similar to planting new seeds in fertile ground.

  - **Release of Growth Factors:**
- Engaging in physical activities increases the secretion of BDNF and other growth factors, essentially fertilizing the brain to support neuronal growth and connectivity.

- **Overall Effects:**
  - **Cognitive Reserve & Brain Health:**
- Combined mental and physical exercises contribute to an increased cognitive reserve, building a buffer against age-related declines analogous to saving funds for a future investment.
- This collaborative effort between mental and bodily engagement not only bolsters overall brain function but also offers a protective shield against neurodegenerative diseases, much like a robust immune system defending against illnesses.

This extensive look at the mechanisms behind brain exercises shows us how interwoven our cognitive and physical routines are in maintaining the vitality of our neural 'garden.' By encouraging a mix of stimulating tasks and vigorous movements, we can nurture a well-rounded and resilient brain capable of incredible adaptability and endurance.

Understanding our brain's neuroplasticity offers an empowering realization: we are equipped with the innate ability to adapt and improve our cognitive functions. No matter the stage of life, the brain retains this dynamic quality, enabling us to master new skills and recover from adversities. By engaging in regular mental and physical exercises, we can actively influence our neural architecture, strengthening it much like a muscle. This knowledge does not just serve as a beacon of hope for those recovering from neurological injuries but also acts as a guide for anyone looking to enhance their mental acuity. Embracing the concept of neuroplasticity is not just about embracing change; it's about taking control of our brain's development and unlocking the full potential of our mental capabilities.

LANGUAGE UNLOCKED THE LINGUISTIC BRAIN

Imagine you're entering a grand library, where each book represents a piece of knowledge. Similarly, this chapter invites you to step into the realm of the linguistic brain, a space where language is not just spoken or heard but intricately processed. Here, we explore how the brain functions as masterfully as a librarian, categorizing and retrieving language with remarkable precision. Understanding this process reveals the brain's extraordinary ability to not only use language but to learn and adapt it, which is critical for everything from forming personal relationships to advancing in one's career. This journey into the linguistic brain will illuminate how we communicate and why that ability is central to our experience as humans.

In the brain, language processing is governed by specialized regions that work together seamlessly, much like different departments within a library. The Broca's area, located in the frontal lobe, is the department responsible for speech production. It orchestrates the movement of muscles to create spoken words, functioning like the library's event organizer planning and executing a successful public reading.

Conversely, the Wernicke's area, found in the temporal lobe, is akin to the library's information desk. It processes the words we hear and read, ensuring comprehension and enabling us to understand the language, like a librarian who helps you find a book you're looking for.

These areas are connected by a neural network that allows for the fluid exchange of information, ensuring that speech and comprehension are coordinated, much as library departments work together to maintain service and order. Understanding the roles that these critical language centers play helps to comprehend how our brains manage the intricate task of language, highlighting the importance of each 'department's' contribution to the efficacy of our daily communication.

When words reach our ears, the journey of understanding and responding begins in the brain's auditory cortex, which recognizes the sounds as language. These signals are then rapidly forwarded to Wernicke's area, the brain's language comprehension center. Much like a receiving department that checks and interprets incoming goods, Wernicke's area deciphers meanings, context, and language nuances.

Once processed, the information travels along a dedicated neural pathway known as the arcuate fasciculus to Broca's area. This specialized route is akin to a private conveyor belt between two departments, ensuring the transfer is swift and direct. Arriving at Broca's area, the fine-tuned coordination comes to fruition. Like the speaking representative of our library, Broca's area organizes thoughts into a sequence of understandable speech, coordinating the vocal cords and mouth muscles to produce words we can share with others.

However, if this network is disrupted, communication breaks down. Damage to Broca's area impairs speech production; words may be slow or slurred, mirroring a disorganized event coordinator in our library analogy. Meanwhile, damage to Wernicke's area affects comprehension. The individual might speak fluently but without coherent meaning, like a misfiled book that's beautifully bound but holds no content. In either case of aphasia, the seamless flow between these areas is fractured, much as a disrupted department in a library hinders overall operation.

Understanding the precise roles of these language centers and their cooperation is key to grasping how our brains orchestrate the remarkable feat of language. This intricate system, remarkably similar to a library's different departments working in tandem, showcases not only the complexity but also the fragility and significance of language processing in our daily lives.

Imagine we're building a house from the ground up, where each stage of construction represents a different phase of language development. First, we lay down the foundation—this is your vocabulary, the collection of words that form the base of language. Just like a strong foundation is crucial to the integrity of a building, a broad vocabulary is essential for robust communication.

Next, we establish the structure using beams and pillars, much like the grammar rules that connect and support the words. Grammar gives sentences their shape and stability, enabling us to construct meaning in the same way that the frame of a house provides it with form and function.

Finally, once our building is sturdy, we adorn it with the finishing touches—paint, trimmings, and decorations. Compare this to sprinkling our conversations with idiomatic expressions and nuanced turns of phrase, the elements that furnish language with personality and color.

In this way, the stages of language development can be understood as constructing a building from scratch. Each stage is crucial and builds upon the last, creating a structure that's not only functional but also a reflection of individual style and cultural identity, much like a well-loved home.

Here is the breakdown of how we build the linguistic blocks that make up our language capabilities, shared in a way that feels like we're unraveling a mystery together over coffee:

- **Vocabulary Acquisition:**
  - Brain's recognition system has a 'filing method' where it matches new words to images or experiences, much like associating a new contact's name with their face.
    - Associative Learning: Connects new words to existing knowledge like a puzzle piece finding its rightful place.
    - Semantic Networking: Organizes words in the brain's 'library' based on meanings and relationships, setting up a map where related words are closer to each other.

- **Grammar Construction:**
  - Our minds follow 'building codes' for correct syntax, stringing words together based on an internal set of grammatical blueprints.
    - Syntax Assembly: Similar to constructing sentences using a LEGO instruction manual that guides which linguistic block goes where.
    - Error-Correction Processes: Acts as a real-time 'grammar checker' during language use, scanning for mistakes and fixing them as we speak or write.

- **Idiomatic and Nuanced Language Use:**
  - The brain gets trained to read between the lines, deciphering nuanced expressions that don't translate directly, akin to understanding the subtext in a novel.
    - Metaphor and Idiom Interpretation: Teaches us to convert figurative expressions into literal understanding, much like decoding a secret message.
    - Cultural and Contextual Understandings: Picks up on the subtle cues

and undertones in language like a sociologist understands a culture's unspoken rules.

Each of these puzzle pieces comes together to grant us the natural ease of using language. They combine the straightforward with the intricate, allowing us to engage in everything from simple daily interactions to crafting stories that captivate the imagination. It's like constructing a home where every brick contributes to the overall integrity and character—a home for the mind that speaks volumes about who we are.

Consider the bilingual brain as an impressive library that houses a vast collection of books in multiple languages. Just as a librarian possesses the skill to organize books by genre and author, the bilingual brain has cognitive strategies for categorizing and retrieving the correct linguistic information.

The brain employs a remarkable cataloging system that allows for separation yet easy access to different language 'sections'. It's akin to the way a librarian uses a master key to move between exclusive sections of a library, each filled with books in different alphabets yet meticulously organized to prevent a mix-up.

When a bilingual speaker switches from one language to another, it's much like the librarian finding and presenting a volume from the right section. This switch involves complex cognitive tasks, including inhibiting one language while activating another – a mental maneuver as swift and seamless as a librarian ensuring the right book is always at hand for the library's patrons.

The ability to manage two languages involves a delicate balance and demonstrates not just the brain's capacity for language but also its incredible adaptability and efficiency. This analogy underscores the sophistication behind the everyday phenomenon of bilingual communication, transforming the concept into a relatable and digestible narrative.

Let's take a deeper look at the bilingual brain's inner workings, where language processing becomes a symphony of complexity and simplicity. Imagine each language like a distinct section in a massive library, complete with its own set of books — that's how our brain houses different language lexicons. These dedicated sections in the brain's library are the temporal and parietal lobes, each equipped to handle the wealth of vocabulary from both languages.

When it's time to speak or understand a language, the brain's librarian — the executive control system — springs into action, deftly navigating through the cerebral catalog and retrieving the correct words or grammar. Like a skilled librarian scanning barcodes, language-specific neurons are activated to access the right section of our neural library.

Language switching, then, is a remarkable feat where this librarian must suppress the noise from one language section while amplifying another, all without disrupting the library's serenity. It's this delicate act of inhibition and activation that allows bilingual individuals to switch languages with the ease of flipping a light switch, gracefully silencing one linguistic flow as the other comes alive.

Further, bilingual brain management relies on executive functions, such as working memory, which keeps track of ongoing conversations, and attention control, which ensures focus amid language overlap. The bilingual 'librarian' within us continuously processes multiple cues, manages tasks, and navigates interruptions, ensuring the library's operation remains smooth and effective.

Understanding these dynamic processes helps to unravel the rich tapestry of the bilingual experience, revealing how managing two languages enriches mental agility and cognitive capabilities. Just like a beautifully run library becomes a beacon of knowledge, the bilingual brain stands as a testament to the wondrous adaptability and potential of the human mind.

Language disorders like aphasia can derail the fluent exchange of words just as a disorganized library causes disruptions in locating information. Aphasia, specifically, occurs when parts of the brain responsible for language are damaged, often due to a stroke or head injury, resulting in difficulties with speaking, understanding, reading, or writing. It's as if the brain's internal library has had its sections jumbled, with the fiction mixed into nonfiction, and reference books scattered all over the place.

The brain works tirelessly to restore order, much like a librarian who must re-catalog and re-shelve books correctly after an upheaval. The reorganization is an arduous process, involving speech therapy to rebuild language skills and regain communication abilities. Notable individuals, like the political strategist James Carville, who experienced transient aphasia, exemplify resilience. Their journeys underscore the possibility of relearning language and the brain's capacity for recovery, even after significant disruption.

In these cases, recalling words or forming coherent sentences can be as challenging as searching for a misplaced book in a library, but with continual reorganization and rehabilitation, the brain can rediscover its linguistic pathways. These stories not only provide insight into the hardships faced by individuals with language disorders but also serve as testimony to the brain's remarkable plasticity and the human spirit's determination.

Let's take a deeper look at the diverse landscape of aphasia, exploring the multifaceted approaches to healing and understanding that mirror the intricate categorization within a vast library. When we speak of non-fluent aphasia, such as Broca's aphasia, we're addressing a type where the flow of speech is halting and laborious; it's comparable to a catalog system that struggles to index new entries efficiently. Meanwhile, fluent aphasia, like Wernicke's, represents a situation where speech remains fluid but loses its meaning, akin to a library where the books are beautifully organized by binding but hold mismatched content.

Speech therapy techniques are as varied as library cataloging systems, tailored to the specific aphasia challenges. For non-fluent aphasias, exercises might focus on rebuilding sentence structure, much like repairing a broken cataloging system. In cases of fluent aphasias, the focus may shift to improving language comprehension, similar to updating a library index for accurate information retrieval.

Neuroplasticity, the brain's remarkable ability to adapt and change, plays a pivotal role in recovering language capabilities. It's as if, after a section of the library has suffered damage, the brain reorganizes its collections, creating new pathways to restore access. This process, much like re-cataloging a library's collections in a new system, takes time, patience, and skill.

Real-life stories of those who have navigated these turbulent waters provide unique insights — take, for example, a politician who, after facing the challenges of non-fluent aphasia, employs strategic pauses and simplified syntax to convey powerful speeches. Or a writer who, despite fluent aphasia, relearns the dance of meaningful dialogue through melody and rhythm exercises.

These individual journeys illuminate the tailored nature of aphasia therapy, demonstrating that language recovery is as personal and varied as the stories within the pages of a library's many books. Through understanding these nuanced pathways to recovery, we gain a deeper appreciation for the complexity and resilience of both the human brain and spirit.

As we've watched libraries transition from the quiet havens of bookshelves into dynamic hubs with digital databases, so too has the way we communicate language been transformed by technology. Just as libraries now offer e-books and online archives, our day-to-day language has morphed to include the quick, abbreviated conversations of texting and the expansive dialogues of social media platforms.

The brain is continually adapting to these new formats of interaction, learning to parse emoji-laden sentences and hashtags with the same ease as it would a well-punctuated letter. It's undertaking an evolution akin to the way a librarian learns to manage electronic records after years of cataloging hard copies. Our neurons are firing in new patterns, forming connections that smooth the transition from traditional to digital communication like librarians seamlessly integrating online systems into their research repertoire.

This technological shift has stretched the boundaries of language, testing our brain's plasticity. Yet, just as efficiently as a modern library system retrieves information with a typed query, our minds now anticipate predictive text inputs and comprehend online shorthand. Revealing language's resilience and our innate ability to adapt, this shift signals not only the progression of human communication but also the astonishing versatility of the human mind.

Let's take a deeper look at how, much like adapting from paper maps to GPS navigation, our brains recalibrate to navigate the language landscape sculpted by technology. When it comes to emojis and online abbreviations, the brain's visual and linguistic centers light up differently compared to traditional text. It's akin to recognizing symbols on a road sign rather than reading a detailed instruction manual — the cognitive load shifts, tapping into more instantaneous, intuitive forms of interpretation.

Reading on screens, the brain orchestrates a different set of neural gymnastics than with paper. Our eyes dart across lit surfaces, sometimes leading to quicker fatigue, much like trying to find your way in bright, unfamiliar territory as opposed to a well-trodden, softly-lit path. This can alter our focus, and evidence suggests that retention can take a hit, as if our brain's 'bookmark' feature doesn't hold as firmly in the digital domain.

As we constantly switch between chat windows, emails, and social feeds, our neurons are wiring new pathways to manage this digital multitasking. Imagine a librarian who used to handle one book at a time now scanning multiple screens at once, tirelessly updating records — that's the level of adaptation our brains are performing.

Socially, the impact is profound. Conversations once held around the dinner table or in office hallways now often take place via quick text exchanges and collaborative online platforms. It compels human interactions to be more brief, more frequent, changing the tempo and rhythm of our social dance. Professional discussions that might have unfolded over days can now be compressed into an email thread completed in hours.

This discourse tours the often unseen cognitive remodelings and social reshufflings that the digital age ushers in. By understanding these shifts, we gather not only the knowledge of how our brains and behaviors are changing but also an appreciation for our capacity to adapt in the face of unceasing technological advancement.

In this chapter, like a library brimming with books, we've explored the brain's vast capabilities for language processing. To understand this complex system is to unlock a deeper level of communication, allowing for a more nuanced exchange of ideas and emotions. The way we learn language, from the basic building of vocabulary to the advanced use of idioms, mirrors the organization and retrieval of information in a library, a testament to the intricate design and function of human cognition. Additionally, witnessing our brain's adaptation to the rapidly evolving technological landscape underscores its remarkable plasticity. This understanding offers us a panoramic view of language's role in our lives, underlining its importance in shaping thoughts, culture, and the essence of human connection. Each insight we have gathered here adds a volume to our personal library of knowledge, enhancing our appreciation for the brain's role as the curator of language and the architect of communication.

SLEEPS MYSTERIES THE SLUMBERING BRAIN

You have now entered "Sleep's Mysteries: The Slumbering Brain," where we unravel the nightly journey our brain undergoes during sleep. This chapter dives into the silent yet critical work of our sleeping minds: restoring energy, consolidating memories, and processing the vast array of information encountered each day. Sleep, an essential function as vital as breathing, plays a pivotal role not only in cognitive health but also in overall physical well-being. By understanding the mechanics and importance of our slumber, we gain insight into how sleep shapes our waking lives, influencing everything from mood regulation to long-term brain health. Join us as we explore the hidden world of sleep and discover its profound impact on our daily existence.

As we lay our heads down at the end of a day, the first stage of sleep greets us like twilight, that serene time when the last rays of the sun brush the horizon. It's a light nap on a lazy Sunday afternoon; easy to wake from but the first step into night's embrace. Diving deeper, we reach a state of true slumber, akin to the quietude of a world blanketed by a late-night snowfall, peaceful and still. This is the restorative sleep that heals and rebuilds. Finally, we enter REM sleep, where the mind's theater comes alive. It is as vivid and active as an audience's imagination in a darkened cinema, with dreams weaving stories out of the day's thoughts and feelings. Each stage of sleep serves a purpose, from the gentle lull of the opening act to the deep, healing interval, and then the grand, dream-filled finale. Together, they compose the nightly symphony that recharges our minds and prepares us for the dawn of a new day.

Here is the breakdown on the indispensable operations our body performs during each stage of sleep, illustrated with analogies to make the science feel as familiar as the comfort of our own beds:

- **Light Sleep (Stage 1 & 2):**
  - **Heart Rate and Body Temperature:**
    - Picture the body like a computer winding down for sleep mode; the heart rate slows and the body cools down, conserving energy for the night ahead.

- **Theta Waves:**
    - Envision radio waves gently humming at a low frequency. Similarly, theta waves indicate the brain is downshifting from the alertness of wakefulness to the calm of early sleep.
- **Role in Transition:**
    - Think of light sleep as the twilight zone of slumber, laying the foundation for the brain and body's descent into the depths of deep sleep.

- **Deep Sleep (Stage 3 & 4):**
    - **Delta Waves:**
        - Much like the deep, resonant tones of a bass guitar, delta waves reverberate through the sleeping brain, signifying that we have entered the restorative powerhouse stage of deep sleep.
    - **Physiological Benefits:**
        - This stage is the overnight repair workshop where the body's maintenance crew comes in; tissue is repaired, vital growth hormones are released, and our internal defense systems are bolstered.

- **REM Sleep:**
    - **Brain Activity:**
        - If our brain activity during REM were a light, it would shine as brightly as during the day. This stage is critical for sifting and storing memories, not unlike a librarian archiving the day's events.
    - **Creativity and Problem-Solving:**
        - It's also the mind's creative studio, bursting with activity that consolidates learning and enhances our ability to come up with novel solutions.

Understanding these steps is akin to learning the secret rhythms of an enchanting nightly dance our bodies perform; each phase choreographed to ensure that we wake refreshed, revitalized, and ready to step into a new day.

The process of falling asleep isn't just about feeling tired; it's a complex biological routine orchestrated by our bodies. As the day winds down, our brain starts to release a hormone called melatonin. You can think of melatonin as the body's natural 'night mode' setting, signaling that it's time to rest. This hormone helps lower our alertness and makes sleep more inviting.

Meanwhile, our brain waves begin to change their rhythm. During waking hours, our brain is abuzz with activity, firing rapid, irregular waves. As we transition towards sleep, these waves start to slow down and synchronize, like the steady drumbeat of a calming song, guiding us into a restful state.

On a deeper level, sleep-inducing processes involve a push-pull dynamic between different brain regions and neurotransmitters, chemicals that carry messages between brain cells. In simple terms, there's a system in the brain that promotes wakefulness, and another that signals when it's time to sleep. When the 'sleep' signals overpower the 'awake' signals, we drift off to sleep.

Understanding these sleep signals and patterns is a bit like figuring out the inner workings of a sophisticated machine. Each component plays a critical role in ensuring we get the rest we need to refresh our minds and bodies for the next day. It's a fascinating interplay of biology that underscores how remarkable, yet methodically, our bodies prepare us for sleep.

As evening darkness envelops the sky, our internal sleep-inducing process kicks into gear. The pineal gland, a pea-sized organ in the brain, starts to secrete melatonin. This hormone doesn't just send a signal; it works in tandem with the suprachiasmatic nucleus, our brain's master clock situated above the point where the optic nerves cross, to control our sleep-wake cycle. This clock is sensitive to light and uses the dimming signals from our eyes as a cue to trigger the release of melatonin, gradually nudging us towards sleepiness.

When our heads hit the pillow and our eyes close, our brain activity begins a remarkable transformation. During the alert hours, it's like a lively symphony with a rapidly-changing score. As we edge closer to slumber, this music begins to slow, the waveforms of our brain's electrical activity elongating into what are known as alpha waves—a prelude to the theta waves of light sleep and the slower delta waves of deep sleep. They guide the brain's descent into the stillness needed for all the restorative work ahead in deep sleep.

Now, let's focus on the molecular messengers of our brain, the neurotransmitters. Imagine GABA and adenosine as the body's natural sleep promoters, encouraging relaxation and drowsiness. GABA acts like a dimmer switch, turning down the brain's arousal levels, while adenosine accumulates the longer we're awake, eventually tipping the scales towards the need for rest. On the flip side, cortisol and adrenaline are like the brain's alarm system, keeping us alert and oriented during our active periods. Their levels drop when it's time to sleep, clearing the stage for GABA and adenosine to take the spotlight.

Within the brain lies an intricate network of sleep and wake centers playing a constant game of tug-of-war. The ventrolateral preoptic nucleus, a group of sleep-inducing neurons, works against the ascending arousal system, which tries to keep us awake. As we prepare for sleep, the VLPO gains the upper hand, suppressing the arousal system and thus reducing sensory input and motor activity, leading us to a tranquil state of unconsciousness.

By understanding these mechanisms, we can appreciate the finely-tuned nature of our sleep-wake regulation, each chemical and neuron playing a pivotal role in the quality and rejuvenation of our sleep, influencing our alertness, mood, and health the next day.

Imagine your brain as a bustling office where the day's work—memories in this analogy—needs to be filed away for later use. During the day, your brain's hippocampus operates like an efficient secretary, taking in the flood of information and quickly deciding where they'll be temporarily stored. But only when we switch off the lights and close the shop for the night, during sleep, does the real organizing happen.

In the still of the night, the brain behaves much like a meticulous night shift worker. It takes every piece of information—each email opened, every conversation had—and begins to sort them. The deeper stages of sleep, particularly REM sleep, are when your brain processes and consolidates these memories, securely transferring them from the hippocampus to more permanent storage in the neocortex, similar to moving documents from 'In Progress' to a 'Saved' file in a well-organized computer.

This nightly process is critical; it's when your brain decides what's important enough to keep and what can be forgotten, akin to a smart email filter that knows exactly which messages to archive for long-term reference and which to send to the trash. By the time you wake up, your 'desk' is clean, and you're ready to take on the new day's information with a clear head. Understanding this hidden nocturnal operation helps us appreciate why good sleep is so vital — it's not just rest for the body but also crucial maintenance for the cognitively demanding tasks we undertake while awake.

Let's take a deeper look at the night shift happening inside our heads as we sleep, the one that's all about solidifying our memories. The neurotransmitter acetylcholine plays a lead role here—it's like the director of neuron activity, deciding which neural pathways will be strengthened based on the day's experiences.

While we're off in dreamland, the hippocampus and the prefrontal cortex are busy having a deep conversation. The hippocampus, which is like a temporary storage for the day's events, passes on information to the prefrontal cortex—where long-term memories are stored. It's kind of like transferring data from a USB drive to a more reliable hard drive for safekeeping.

Now, in the REM stage of sleep, our brains start to 'tidy up' by pruning the synaptic connections. Think of it like editing your work—cutting out the extraneous bits to leave only the crispest, clearest memories behind. It's a careful process of deciding which memories are keepers and which can be let go.

Lastly, during the slow-wave sleep phase, our brains are like athletes in a quiet practice session, going over the movements learned throughout the day without actually moving. This is when procedural memories, which are related to skills and tasks, get ingrained. So, if you're learning to play the piano or mastering a new tennis serve, it's during this time that your brain cements what your muscles should remember, all while you're sound asleep.

Through this intricate interplay of chemicals, synapses, and brain waves, every night sets the stage for the memories that help us navigate life. It's this extraordinary phenomenon that turns fleeting moments into long-lasting learnings, proving that a good night's sleep is a prolific part of our learning and memory process.

Sleep disorders are a group of conditions that disrupt the quality, timing, or duration of sleep, impacting daily life. Insomnia, for example, is the difficulty in falling or staying asleep. It's like lying in bed with a switched-on mind that refuses to power down. Then there's sleep apnea, which causes pauses in breathing during sleep, much like a stuttering engine that hinders a car's smooth run. Restless legs syndrome gives an uncontrollable urge to move the legs, a feeling akin to an incessant phone vibration that you cannot ignore. Narcolepsy leads to overwhelming drowsiness and sudden sleep attacks, similar to your phone battery suddenly dropping to zero percent.

These disturbances can have profound consequences, from diminished alertness to severe health issues, much like how a device's performance falters if it's not charged properly. Arianna Huffington, the co-founder of The Huffington Post, realized the seriousness of sleep deprivation after a wake-up call: she collapsed from exhaustion. Since then, she's become an advocate for taking sleep seriously, showing that even the most driven individuals are not immune to its effects.

Understanding sleep disorders is key to acknowledging their potential side effects and recognizing the importance of seeking proper treatment. It highlights a universal truth: sleep is not just a period of inactivity but a critical function as impactful on our health as diet and exercise.

Let's take a deeper look at the intricate biological underpinnings of sleep disorders and demystify the paths to their diagnosis and treatments, drawing parallels to everyday experiences to elucidate the subject.

Chronic insomnia often stems from factors such as unyielding stress, analogous to a persistent background noise that disrupts focus, or from habits detrimental to sleep, like a phone screen's blue light tricking our brain's clock into wakefulness. To untangle the roots of insomnia, doctors delve into a patient's sleep history, akin to a detective piecing together clues. They may also conduct a sleep study, where the patient's nighttime patterns are observed and recorded, looking for disruptions as revealing as unexpected plot twists in a novel.

With sleep apnea, imagine a narrow mountain pass that becomes blocked by falling rocks, halting traffic flow—that's what happens in the throat during sleep apnea episodes, as the muscles there relax and obstruct breathing. Doctors use a polysomnography test, an overnight recording session that monitors various body functions during sleep, functioning like a surveillance system to detect and confirm this blockage.

Restless legs syndrome involves an internal imbalance of dopamine, a neurotransmitter that acts much like a gear oil, ensuring the smooth movement of muscle machinery. If off-balance, patients may feel an uncomfortable sensation urging leg movements. Diagnosing this syndrome involves taking thorough medical histories and conducting physical exams to identify its puzzling symptoms accurately.

The insidious culprit in narcolepsy is often an orexin deficiency. Orexin, a chemical messenger as crucial for wakefulness as a pilot in a cockpit, when it's deficient, the ability to stay awake plummets drastically. Diagnosing narcolepsy includes specific tests like the multiple sleep latency test, wherein short naps are monitored throughout the day to measure the speed of falling asleep, as telling as the response time of emergency services.

Treatment options might include behavior modification, like establishing soothing nighttime rituals similar to setting the stage for an evening performance. Medications can be as specific as tuning an instrument for optimal performance, while lifestyle changes, like diet and exercise, are akin to general rehearsal, each contributing to the symphony of a good night's rest.

By comprehending these details, one can navigate the complexities of sleep disorders with clarity, recognizing the importance of tailored approaches to restore the harmony of restful sleep.

In conclusion, "Sleep's Mysteries: The Slumbering Brain" has illuminated the nightly voyage our brains undertake to rejuvenate and reorganize. We've uncovered how sleep stages are essential for memory consolidation, the pivotal role of melatonin and brain waves in ushering in rest, and how sleep disorders can disrupt this delicate balance with significant consequences. We've seen the brain's remarkable nightly rejuvenation from bustling neural activity to the silent, healing pause of deep sleep, reinforcing the critical nature of sleep for cognitive function and overall health. This exploration has highlighted that sleep is not a passive state but an active and dynamic process crucial for maintaining our mental acuity and well-being. The revelations from this chapter are a call to acknowledge and prioritize sleep, empowering us with the knowledge to enhance our life's quality and longevity.

NAVIGATING THE MAZE STROKE AND RECOVERY

Strokes are depicted as blockages in a city's water supply, exploring how interruptions in blood flow affect the brain and the journey to recovery.

In "Navigating the Maze: Stroke and Recovery," we address the sudden and often devastating impact of stroke on the brain, drawing a parallel to an unexpected and severe storm that disrupts a city's workings. The chapter will guide readers through the aftermath, shedding light on the acute challenges a stroke presents and the subsequent recovery process. Focusing on the mechanisms of the brain affected by stroke, the road to regaining lost functions, and the significant role of rehabilitative therapies, this chapter aims to provide a clear understanding of stroke's effects and the strategies used to navigate the road to recovery. By examining this journey, we aim to offer valuable insights into the resilience of the human brain and the critical steps required to rebuild and adapt after such life-altering events.

Strokes come in two major types: ischemic and hemorrhagic. An ischemic stroke is like a blockage occurring in a highway that disrupts traffic flow. It happens when a clot blocks a blood vessel in the brain, stopping blood and oxygen from reaching brain cells, which can cause them to die. This is the most common stroke type and can lead to difficulties with movement or speech, depending on which brain area is affected.

On the other hand, a hemorrhagic stroke is similar to a water pipe bursting, causing flooding and damage. This type of stroke takes place when a weakened blood vessel in the brain ruptures and bleeds into the surrounding brain tissue. The bleeding causes swelling and increased pressure, leading to damage or irritation of the brain cells in that area. The symptoms can be similar to an ischemic stroke but may also include a sudden headache or loss of consciousness.

Both types of strokes have a significant impact on the brain's functionality. They can affect movement, speech, vision, and cognition because they disrupt the normal blood flow in critical areas of the brain that control these functions. Understanding the differences between these strokes is essential because it determines the medical approach to treat them and the recovery process. The goal is clear: to either remove the blockage in an ischemic stroke or reduce the bleeding and pressure in a hemorrhagic stroke, thus minimizing brain damage and improving the chances of recovery.

When dealing with an ischemic stroke, time is of the essence. Clot-busting drugs like tPA (tissue plasminogen activator) must be administered typically within a four-and-a-half-hour window after stroke symptoms begin. This drug works to dissolve the clot that's obstructing blood flow to the brain. In some cases, a mechanical thrombectomy, which involves physically removing the clot using a specialized device threaded through an artery, can be performed. This procedure is generally most effective if done within six to twenty-four hours of the onset of symptoms.

For hemorrhagic strokes, surgical intervention may be needed to reduce intracranial pressure—this involves making a small hole in the skull to drain accumulated blood and reduce the pressure on the brain. Other times, aneurysm repair procedures, such as clipping or coiling, are used to stop the bleeding. It's also crucial to manage and monitor blood pressure to prevent further vessel damage.

Rehabilitation is a tailored process that addresses the specific deficits left by the stroke. Physical therapy helps patients regain strength and coordination. Speech therapy works on improving language and swallowing difficulties. Occupational therapy assists with relearning daily activities and tasks.

An example of a day in rehabilitation might include a morning spent with physical therapists working on balance and walking, followed by sessions with a speech therapist practicing speaking and comprehension tasks, and in the afternoon, occupational therapy to work on skills like dressing or cooking.

Throughout recovery, a multidisciplinary team that includes neurologists, rehabilitation therapists, nurses, and social workers, among others, collaborate to create a detailed care plan. This plan is focused on helping the stroke survivor regain as much independence as possible and ultimately improve their quality of life.

In the critical moments of a stroke, medical teams spring into action with the immediacy and coordinated effort you'd expect from first responders to a natural disaster. Picture an emergency crew swiftly assessing the situation and determining the best course of action—this is what doctors do when they're evaluating a stroke. Using rapid imaging tests, such as a CT scan, as their reconnaissance, they're able to locate the 'storm center' of the stroke. Much like deciding on evacuations or immediate repairs during a catastrophe, doctors quickly choose the most effective treatment. If a clot has caused the stroke, a clot-busting drug may be administered, acting like emergency services working to clear a blocked road. In the case of a bleed, doctors work urgently to stabilize the patient to prevent more damage, similar to how emergency measures are taken to reinforce a damaged dam. This intricate dance of decisive movements is guided by the singular goal to prevent extensive fallout and to rescue as many 'inhabitants'—in this case, brain cells—as possible.

Here is the breakdown of the critical initial response to a stroke, laid out in a way that brings clarity to a high-stakes situation:

- **Initial Assessment:**
    - On arrival at the hospital, imagine the medical team as a pit crew in a race, where speed and precision are crucial. They quickly check the patient's 'engine vitals', such as blood pressure and heart rate.
    - Specialists perform a neurological examination, akin to running a system diagnostic, checking for areas of impairment.
    - There's an urgency to estimate stroke severity, with scales like the NIHSS acting similar to a storm scale, assessing the damage severity and potential impact.

- **Diagnostic Imaging:**
    - CT scans or MRIs act like high-definition satellite images, giving doctors a clear 'aerial view' of where and what the 'storm'—the stroke—looks like.
    - Interpretation of these images determines the type of stroke, whether it's caused by a 'roadblock' or a 'burst pipeline'—ischemic or hemorrhagic.

- **Treatment Decision:**
    - For ischemic stroke:
        - Administering tPA is like dispatching a specialized 'clean-up crew' to dissolve the blockage, but it's time-sensitive, typically within 4.5 hours of

symptom onset.
- Assessment of any reasons the patient might not be able to receive tPA to avoid causing more harm than good.
- For hemorrhagic stroke:
- Options may include surgical procedures, like clipping or coiling—analogous to repair workers fixing a burst water main to stop further flooding.
- An evacuation of hematoma to reduce pressure in the brain, much like clearing debris after a landslide to prevent additional damage.

- **Stabilization:**
- After the initial 'storm' passes, the next phase is like rebuilding a town to prevent future calamities.
- Controlling blood pressure is like reinforcing the levees, ensuring they don't give way again.
- Management of brain swelling, comparable to providing disaster relief to prevent after-effects.
- Continuous monitoring is akin to a weather station keeping a vigilant eye for aftershocks or secondary storms.

- **Multidisciplinary Team Deployment:**
- Roles vary from neurologists, who are the 'architects' of the intervention plan, to emergency physicians, who are the 'first responders' assessing and managing immediate risks, to stroke nurses, who work as the hands and feet on the ground, vigilantly implementing the care plan.

By piecing together these finely tuned steps, this detailed explanation illustrates the sensitivity and complexity of stroke care. It shows that every action taken is part of a larger strategy aiming to minimize damage and set the stage for recovery—much like a community comes together in a concerted effort to mend and rebuild after a devastating natural disaster.

Think of stroke rehabilitation as the meticulous restoration of a historical town after an unforeseen calamity. The process unfolds in stages: emergency work to stabilize the structures, careful planning for reconstruction, and the hard toil of rebuilding, all with the hope of returning to former glory or perhaps achieving a new, adapted state of normalcy.

First comes the need for stability—akin to swiftly erecting scaffolds around weakened buildings. Here, patients might work in early mobility therapy to prevent muscle weakness and maintain circulation, such as sitting up, standing, or even walking, depending on their condition.

Then, the blueprint of recovery is drawn; goals are set much like a town planner would design a revitalization project. Specific therapies are the tools of reconstruction. Physical therapy helps rebuild the muscles and nerves' pathways, akin to the repair of roads and bridges, enabling the patient to regain movement and dexterity. Occupational therapy revolves around the daily essentials, resembling the restoration of town services, ensuring patients can navigate day-to-day life effectively. Speech therapy focuses on communication capabilities, quite like the repair of communication lines, to ensure that patients can express their needs and thoughts.

Throughout this period, milestones are celebrated; each small victory is a brick in the wall, a signpost of progress. The ability to move a limb or articulate a word can be as momentous as the reopening of a town square, heralding a return to communal life.

This journey is intensive and requires a team as dedicated as any community of builders, engineers, and volunteers. It's a testament to the tenacity of both stroke survivors and the professionals who guide them towards reclaiming their autonomy, crafting from the debris a life reshaped yet resilient.

Let's take a deeper look at the purposeful activities and benchmarks that punctuate the journey of stroke rehabilitation, much akin to tracking the progress of a city's reconstruction, brick by brick:

- **Physical Therapy:**
    - Range-of-motion Activities: These are like the foundational groundwork after a disaster, helping to prevent stiffness and gradual loss of function by moving the joints gently through their full span.
    - Strength Training: Consider this akin to rebuilding the framework of damaged structures, focusing on fortifying muscle power to improve overall movement and stability.
    - Walking or Gait Training: Tailoring this to individuals is like paving customized pathways for residents to navigate the city, where each path is designed to suit unique mobility needs, ensuring confident and safe traversal.

- **Occupational Therapy:**
  - Self-care Skills: Training in activities like dressing or cooking mirrors the restoration of essential services in a town, making sure citizens can manage their daily needs efficiently.
  - Use of Adaptive Equipment: Introducing tools such as grab bars or extended reachers can be likened to implementing new technologies in the town for greater accessibility and self-sufficiency.
  - Cognitive Rehabilitation: Focused on reviving cognitive functions such as memory, akin to rebooting a town's power grid, enabling restored problem-solving and attentive proficiency in the community.

- **Speech Therapy:**
  - Language Exercises: Here, the rebuilding is of the communication channels, establishing clear lines again through speech improvement practices tailored to individual impairments.
  - Swallowing Therapy: Managing dysphagia relates to ensuring the waterways of the town are clear and flowing correctly, reducing the risk of further complications.

- **Milestone Tracking:**
  - Functional Scales such as the Barthel Index: Imagine these as the inspector's checklists, ensuring each restoration phase meets the set health and safety standards.
  - Outcome Measures like the Fugl-Meyer Assessment: These work like progress reviews to chart the extent of recovery, determining how close the city is to achieving its revitalization goals.

By understanding the nuance in these treatments and regularly marking progress, we map out a stroke survivor's road to recovery with clarity. This detailed view of rehabilitation activities illustrates the commitment to regaining independence, much like a city's dedication to rising again, more robust, and more resilient.

Stroke recovery is a complex process that hinges on the careful adaptation to new challenges and sturdy support systems. It involves not just the patient, but a coordinated squad of healthcare professionals who guide and facilitate rehabilitation, akin to a team of expert coaches. The roles are diverse – from physical therapists who help patients rebuild strength and coordination to speech therapists who assist in regaining communication abilities.

Beyond the professionals, recovery utilizes an array of tools designed to help restore independence. These range from simple devices like canes and grabbers, which can be seen as the recovery equivalents of training wheels, to high-tech equipment like computer programs that aid cognitive therapy.

Personal support networks are another pillar of stroke recovery. Family members, friends, and support groups offer the crucial emotional backing needed, not unlike the rooting section at a sports event, cheering and providing motivation for every small win on the path back to normalcy.

Each of these elements plays a crucial role in navigating the challenging road to recovery. Together, they forge a system as intricate and dependable as any well-functioning community, tailored to foster the comeback journey of someone who has suffered a stroke, aiming to restore as much autonomy and quality of life as possible.

Let's take a deeper look at the concerted efforts of healthcare professionals, the tools they wield like master craftspeople, and the network of support akin to a community coming together after an event shakes its core:

- **For Healthcare Professionals:**
- Occupational therapists act as the architects of daily life, mapping out restoration plans with precision. They assess a patient's abilities to perform activities of daily living, drafting personalized plans that may range from dressing to managing finances.
- Physical therapists are the hands-on builders, guiding patients through exercises that lay the foundation for regained strength. Their tools are stretches to reclaim range of motion and intricate drills that retrain the fine motor skills used for tasks like writing or buttoning shirts.
- Speech therapists serve as the communicators, assessing how well patients can speak and understand others. They develop personalized regimens – speech drills for those with slurred speech (dysarthria) and language exercises for those searching for the right words (aphasia).

- **Tools and Technology in Therapy:**
- Envision a toolkit brimming with aids like button hooks, specially angled utensils, and non-slip mats – simple yet transformative devices that

make the ordinary activities of eating and dressing manageable once again for patients.

- Within the digital world, software for cognitive therapy might include memory games that function like personalized brain teasers, designed to strengthen a patient's ability to recall and use information in everyday situations.

- **Support Networks:**
- Family and friends are the emotional scaffolding offering not only cheers from the sidelines but the assistive hands that help navigate the daily landscape of recovery, from ensuring transportation to therapy sessions to modifying the home environment for safety.
- The safety nets of community services and social work stretch far and wide, providing everything from counseling services to adaptive equipment loans, just as a community center offers varied resources to meet the diverse needs of its members.

Through understanding each of these roles and tools, a clearer picture emerges. Each activity, device, and support person is a thread woven into the larger tapestry of stroke rehabilitation, driving toward a common goal of reintegration into the life that was, or building anew, the life that is still possible.

The recovery narratives of public figures like Arizona Representative Gabrielle Giffords and actor Kirk Douglas serve as powerful showcases of human resilience in the face of adversity. Giffords, after surviving a gunshot wound to the head, had to relearn how to speak and walk, demonstrating immense determination throughout her extensive therapy. Douglas, who survived a stroke at the age of 80, worked tirelessly to regain his speech and went on to continue his acting and writing career. These stories highlight not only personal strength and persistence but also the potential for remarkable recovery with adequate support and rehabilitative care. The journeys of these public figures reinforce the message that, although the path to recovery can be arduous, the human capacity to overcome and adapt is formidable.

Imagine a town, once tranquil, now bustling with construction as it embraces modern refurbishments, from newly paved roads to state-of-the-art buildings. This transformation is akin to the changes unfolding in stroke recovery, thanks to cutting-edge medical technologies. Robotic exoskeletons, for instance, are similar to advanced cranes and machinery, empowering patients to regain movement by providing support as they relearn to walk.

Similarly, virtual reality systems offer immersive environments that help individuals practice real-life tasks; they are like simulations used by urban planners, enabling practice runs and adjustments before the actual execution. Brain-computer interfaces, which translate neural activity into commands for computers or prosthetics, mirror a town's upgrade to a smart-city interface, improving communication and functionality. These innovations provide new roads to recovery that once seemed like science fiction, demonstrating the incredible progress that has been made and opening up more possibilities for stroke survivors to regain independence and improve their quality of life.

Here is the breakdown of the latest technological assistances boosting stroke recovery, akin to the specialized tools that bring an architect's blueprint to life:

- **Robotic Exoskeletons:**
    - These advanced devices are equipped with sensors that detect muscle activity and motors that assist with limb movement, much like a dance partner who supports and follows your lead during rehabilitation exercises.
    - Exoskeletons can be used for gait training, where they provide the necessary support and correction, gently guiding the patient's legs in a walking motion. They keep a digital log of movement patterns and improvements, offering a tangible measure of progress.

- **Virtual Reality Systems:**
    - Patients engage with a variety of simulated tasks that mirror real-life activities, from picking up groceries to maneuvering through crowded spaces, enabling practice in a safe, controlled environment.
    - These systems offer real-time feedback, adjusting the difficulty and assistance level as needed, just as a driving instructor might modulate the challenge of a lesson to match a student's skills.

- **Brain-Computer Interfaces:**
    - By capturing the brain's electrical activity, these sophisticated interfaces can translate thoughts into actions by commanding computers or prosthetics. It's like telepathy with a machine—thinking about moving a digital object on screen and the system responding in kind.
    - Through these interfaces, patients can practice simple actions such as moving a cursor, which can feel like turning the keys of a new car for the first time, hinting at independence and reconnection with the environment.

These technological inventors, much like skilled craftspeople, contribute uniquely to the grand project of recovery. By pinpointing and mapping out each technology's role, we can better understand how they reinforce the journey from patient effort to functional success, offering new avenues to regaining independence after a stroke.

As 'Navigating the Maze: Stroke and Recovery' comes to a close, we reflect on the incredible journey that stroke survivors embark upon, marked by extraordinary resilience and adaptability. Through personal dedication and the support of medical professionals, technology, and community, individuals facing the aftermath of a stroke have the potential to restore their lives in new and meaningful ways. This process echoes the determined efforts of a town rebuilding after devastation, where every step forward is a testament to human strength and the profound ability of people to rise above challenges. This chapter underscores the significance of each individual's path, honoring the complexity of recovery and the indomitable spirit that fuels it, proving that with perseverance and the right support, regaining independence and well-being is within reach.

THE SENSORY TAPESTRY INTERPRETING THE WORLD

The human sensory system is a collective network of bio-scouts, each specialized in specific modes of perception — sight, hearing, taste, smell, and touch — that gather data from our environment. These scouts report back to our brain, which acts as a central command center, decoding and synthesizing the information to shape our understanding of the world around us. This system guides our interaction with our surroundings, influences decision-making, and enables us to experience the richness of life. The impact of these sensory informants extends beyond mere perception; they influence our emotions, memories, and even our communication with others. This chapter introduces the intricate dance of sensory input and neural processing, setting a foundation for discussing the remarkable ways in which our brains interpret complex signals to construct the reality we experience daily.

The journey of sensory information begins at our sensory organs, which are akin to frontline detectors, each attuned to a specific type of stimulus. Take the eyes, for instance, they capture light and translate it into a format suitable for the brain, much as a camera converts a scene into a digital file. This transformation occurs when the light stimulates the retina's photoreceptor cells that, in turn, generate nerve impulses. These impulses are the body's version of electrical signals. From the retina, these signals travel along the optic nerve, a biological data cable, to the brain's visual processing center.

Similarly, each of our other senses — from the vibrations captured by the tiny structures in our ears, to the chemicals detected by our taste buds and scent receptors, to the pressure and temperature discerned by our skin — converts real-world information into nerve impulses. These impulses are the currency of the nervous system, allowing for communication within the brain's complex network.

Once these electrical signals reach the brain, they are processed by specialized regions responsible for interpreting each sense. In the brain's cerebral cortex, the signals from our sensory organs are decoded, analyzed, and interwoven into the single, seamless perception of our surroundings we experience. It's a bit like an orchestra's conductor receiving music from different instruments and blending them into a harmonious symphony. This process allows us to react and interact with our environment in real-time, grounding abstract sensory data into the vivid, tangible world we know.

In the visual pathway, the journey begins with phototransduction, where photons of light hitting the cells in the retina trigger a chemical change in photoreceptors called rods and cones. These cells then alter their output of neurotransmitters, signaling to nearby bipolar cells, which in turn adjust their own signals to the next set of cells, the ganglion cells. Ganglion cells have long axons that bundle together to form the optic nerve, serving as transmission lines sending the visual information straight to the brain. Once in the brain, these signals travel to the lateral geniculate nucleus (LGN) of the thalamus, which acts as a relay center, and then on to the primary visual cortex. Here the raw data is processed to form coherent images, recognizing patterns, edges, colors, and movements.

In the auditory pathway, sound waves are captured by the ear and converted into mechanical vibrations by the eardrum and middle ear bones. These vibrations reach the cochlea, where they cause movement in specific hair cells tuned to different frequencies. When these hair cells move, they generate nerve impulses that travel along the auditory nerve. The signal then proceeds to the cochlear nucleus, which begins to process the timing and intensity of sounds. Next stops include the superior olivary complex, which helps to localize sound, and the inferior colliculus, which refines auditory signals, before reaching the auditory cortex where the brain perceives and interprets the complex symphony of sounds.

Gustatory (taste) information begins at the taste buds, which detect dissolved chemicals as taste. These signals are sent to the brainstem and then to the thalamus before reaching the gustatory cortex, where they are perceived as specific tastes. Olfactory (smell) information involves odorant molecules binding to receptors in the nasal cavity, causing nerve impulses that travel to the olfactory bulb. The olfactory bulb processes the signal and sends it to different brain regions, including the olfactory cortex. The integration of olfactory and gustatory signals is crucial in the overall perception of flavor, allowing us to discern and enjoy the full range of flavors in our meals.

The tactile pathway captures touch, pressure, and vibration through mechanoreceptors in the skin. These receptors transform physical stimulation into nerve impulses, which then follow nerve fibers to the spinal cord, and onward to the somatosensory cortex of the brain. This process allows us to detect a hug's warmth, the pressure of a handshake, and the texture of an object. Different types of mechanoreceptors respond to varying stimuli strengths and durations, enabling a wide spectrum of tactile experiences.

By following the path from sensory receptor to brain interpretation, we obtain a detailed portrayal of how our sensory systems translate the external world into the internal language of the brain, forming our perception of reality.

Neural processing, the brain's method of making sense of the information our senses pick up, begins in the sensory areas of the cortex – specialized departments for each sense. When light hits your eyes or a sound waves reach your ears, it's your sensory areas that get the first crack at decoding what this information could mean. Imagine a mail room in a large company, sorting all incoming packages according to where they're needed.

From here, the information moves onto other regions of the brain where it's scrutinized further – it's sent to the right departments to deal with specifics, like recognising faces or understanding words. Each piece of information, whether a sound, a smell, or touch, is passed along on a need-to-know basis, with more complex processing happening at every step.

Ultimately, this information reaches the higher-order brain centers – the decision-makers. They take all the sorted and analyzed information to form a comprehensive understanding. Think of this like a board meeting where all department heads come together, bringing their reports to formulate a complete picture of the company's status. This 'big picture' is the reality we experience. It's complex, with many hands on deck and several steps, but in essence, it's about getting the raw data, figuring out what it means, and then fitting it all together into an experience that makes sense to us.

Let's take a deeper look at the cellular workers and the neural structures that craft our sensory experiences:

Neurons, the cells that carry messages throughout the nervous system, have unique properties tailored for their signaling role. Picture them as messengers on a delivery route: they have long extensions called axons, which are like express highways for electrical signals, and dendrites, akin to a series of small roads gathering information to be sent out. Each neuron is insulated by a substance called myelin, similar to the rubber coating on wires, ensuring messages aren't lost during transmission.

The thalamus, sitting near the center of the brain, acts as an essential sorting center—a train station of sorts—where sensory messages are redirected to appropriate destinations. It's a relay for the majority of sensory inputs, engaged in preliminary processing like filtering out unnecessary noise or enhancing crucial signals before sending them to the cortex for detailed analysis.

The cortex is the brain's version of a high-tech lab, where sensory information mingles with your memories, and learned knowledge. Association areas, the scientists of the brain, take this raw data, compare it with previous experiences, and color it with emotions to create our moment-to-moment reality. They're essential for making sense of the sensory puzzle, determining, for instance, that the scent wafting through the air is from a rose garden associated with memories of past springs.

High-order brain centers, akin to a seasoned editor, have the ability to modulate incoming sensory signals, highlighting some inputs and muting others, crafting a streamlined narrative. This process is crucial when focusing, for example, tuning out background chatter to concentrate on a conversation at a noisy party.

Lastly, the brain's adaptability, or plasticity, can be likened to a city's ever-evolving map. As you experience the world—learning new skills, encountering new sensations—your brain's connections remap, with busy routes becoming more established and lesser-used paths fading. This adaptability ensures that learning and memory shape how we experience the sensory world.

Understanding these components deepens our appreciation for the intricate interplay that underpins our sensory perceptions. It's a complex system orchestrated with the precision of a symphony, allowing us to navigate and enjoy the richness of the world around us.

Consider how a meal engages all your senses: You see the colorful presentation on the plate, you smell the aromatic spices, you taste the complex flavors, you hear the crunch as you take a bite, and you feel the texture of the food. Each of these sensory inputs is like an instrument in an orchestra, playing its own part. The brain acts as the conductor, expertly blending these separate sensory notes into the symphony of your eating experience.

Each sensory signal enters the brain's concert hall through its own doorway, like musicians arriving from different entrances. Sight, smell, taste, sound, and touch each have their own sections in the brain's orchestra, and each signal comes with its own timbre and pitch. The strength and timing of these signals are fine-tuned, much like how a conductor raises their baton to cue the strings or signal the brass to soften.

The real magic happens when these individual parts are weaved together for the performance, creating a symphony that is far more immersive and comprehensive than any solo act. This integration ensures that what you see complements what you taste and smell, creating a unified sensory feast. Through this collaborative process, where the separate sensations become one, we experience the full pleasure of a meal, which is far more than just the sum of its parts.

Here is the breakdown of the multi-sensory feast we undergo when indulging in a meal, detailed to help us appreciate every nuanced element that our brain harmonizes:

- **Visual Processing:**
    - Light from the attractive dish strikes the retina, where it's captured by photoreceptor cells—our body's personal cameramen.
    - This visual information is sent via the optic nerve, like a fast-track delivery route, to the primary visual cortex at the back of the brain.
    - Here, and in adjoining secondary visual areas, the brain analyzes color and motion, fine-tuning the image as an art critic would inspect a painting's details.

- **Olfactory Pathway:**
  - Scent molecules drift to the nose, docking on receptors like keys in locks, triggering a cascade of neural messages.
  - These messages are wired directly to the olfactory bulb, a hub that processes scent information before relaying it to the brain's olfactory cortex.
  - This is where scents are identified, creating a linkage to memories, emotions, and, importantly, taste perceptions, much like how a fragrance can evoke a specific time or place.

- **Gustatory Processing:**
  - Taste buds, our mouth's own taste testers, recognize and respond to the meal's flavors, sending signals through the cranial nerves.
  - These impulses are forwarded to the gustatory cortex, which decodes them into tastes we recognize—sweet, sour, salty, bitter, and umami.
  - There's a collaborative dialogue with olfactory signals here, as both taste and smell intertwine to produce the full profile of a flavor.

- **Auditory Processing:**
  - The crunch of crispy vegetables or the sizzle from a hot pan is captured by the ears and transformed into vibrations.
  - These vibrations travel through various ear structures and are finally converted into nerve signals that the auditory cortex interprets as recognizable sounds.

- **Somatosensory Processing:**
  - Our skin and oral cavity have tactile receptors that register the textures and temperatures of food, similar to our hands gauging the feel of different materials.
  - Signals from these receptors map to the somatosensory cortex, informing us if the meal is hot, cold, smooth, or crunchy.

- **Multisensory Integration:**
  - The insular cortex acts as a meeting room where all sensory modalities come together to form a cohesive dining experience.
  - Here, the brain integrates the meal's appearance, aroma, taste, sound, and texture into a single, delightful sensory package, much like combining ingredients to create a perfect dish.

This complex coordination ensures that a meal is not just a mere act of eating, but an immersive event to be savored and remembered. Understanding these sensory contributions elucidates the brain's role in shaping our culinary enjoyment and the richness it brings to our lives.

Just as two people might stand before a painting and interpret its story differently, each person's brain processes sensory information in a unique way, leading to personal perceptions of the same environment. Consider how viewers might respond to a piece of abstract art: One might see a chaotic blend of colors, while another detects a hidden message in its patterns. This variation occurs because individual brains—like art critics—focus on and analyze different aspects based on their own experiences and neural wiring.

The brain filters and gives priority to different sensory data, and these preferences shape our conscious experience. For some, colors may appear more vibrant, which could be compared to how a foodie savors the subtle flavors in a dish that others might miss. Memories, too, color our perception, much as a familiar scent might remind one person of home, yet mean little to someone else.

These perceptual differences are the result of the brain's personalized processing routine. Just like art, where each piece speaks differently to its viewers, reality is subject to interpretation. The brain's individualized production of perception is what makes our experiences of the world distinct and rich—an impressive reminder that each person lives in a sensory realm of their own making.

Sommeliers and perfumers possess highly tuned sensory skills that distinguish them in their fields. A sommelier can detect nuanced flavors in wine that might escape the average drinker. This capability isn't just good taste; it's a result of rigorous training and a refined olfactory system. Their brains have honed the ability to pick up and interpret subtle differences in scent and taste. Likewise, perfumers can distinguish between hundreds of scents. They spend years training their noses, memorizing different fragrance profiles, much like a musician must learn to recognize and reproduce a wide range of notes.

The neural mechanisms behind these abilities involve both keen sensory receptors and extensive neural processing. Enhanced wiring in brain areas dedicated to smell and taste, such as the olfactory bulb and the gustatory cortex, allow for the heightened discrimination of flavors and scents. Furthermore, the brain's plasticity plays a role; just as a bodybuilder develops muscles with training, sommeliers and perfumers develop neural pathways with practice.

These professionals also benefit from an extensive 'scent or flavor vocabulary,' allowing them to tag and retrieve scent or taste memories. With each new experience, they build a library of sensory experiences that they can recall and compare against, which is crucial for identifying and describing sensory qualities in their work.

Let's take a deeper look at how sommeliers and perfumers master their exceptional olfactory potential:

Sommeliers often start by inhaling a curated selection of essential wine aromas from specialized kits, much like an athlete runs through a structured workout to improve performance. Daily, they nose through these scents, which might range from fruits to earthy undertones, training their senses to recognize and recall each distinct aroma.

Perfumers, on the other hand, undergo a similar routine, methodically sniffing an array of scent vials. Like learning vocabulary in a new language, they imprint these fragrances into memory through repetition and association. Flashcards of scents, if you will.

These practices are supported by the remarkable ability of their brains to adapt and change—neuroplasticity in action. As a music student learns to play an instrument, creating stronger connections between neurons with each practice session, repeated exposure to specific scents and flavors strengthens the perceptual pathways in these professionals' brains.

Intricate recognition patterns are formed in regions like the hippocampus, the brain's librarian, which archives each scent and taste experience for future retrieval. It's not just about picking up a smell or taste; it's about linking it to a vast internal database of sensory memories, which can be accessed and added to over time.

Developing a robust 'scent or flavor vocabulary' is an integral part of the process, turning a novice into a connoisseur. This vocabulary allows them to identify nuances and communicate about them with precision—akin to a poet finding the perfect words to describe a scene.

Through this deep dive into their routine, we gain insight into the meticulous world of these sensory specialists. We understand the agility and commitment behind each sniff and sip, the neuroscientific choreography that enables them to discern layers of complexity in wine and perfume that elevate their craft to an art form.

The brain's capacity to adapt is akin to a community's resilience in rebuilding after a devastating natural disaster. Just as townspeople come together to restore what was lost, finding new ways to re-establish their lives and livelihoods, our brains can reroute functions and forge new connections in response to sensory loss. If, for instance, someone's vision is impaired, the brain doesn't just accept this change; it starts remodeling, strengthening other senses like hearing or touch, much like a community might repurpose a space to fit a new need. This remarkable flexibility, known as neuroplasticity, showcases the brain's indefatigable spirit to recover and even improve its operations, ensuring that an individual can continue to experience life fully, despite challenges. Just as a town strikes back with newfound strength and unity, the brain compensates for loss by tapping into its innate ability to regenerate and adapt.

Here is the breakdown of the intricate ballet of neuroplasticity, revealed through the lens of everyday miracles:

- **Neuronal Adaptation:**
  - Like adjusting to a sudden change in lighting, neurons recalibrate their responses when sensory inputs are lost, redefining their role in signal transmission.
  - Synapse strengthening, akin to reinforcing a muscle through exercise, and the creation of new synapses, comparable to forging a new path through a forest, enhance the brain's ability to reroute functions effectively.

- **Molecular Mechanisms:**
  - Neurotrophic factors, the brain's growth fertilizers, are released to nurture neuron survival and encourage the outgrowth of new connections.
  - Neurotransmitters, the chemical messengers of the brain, akin to postal

workers delivering mail, become vital in establishing these nascent pathways and ensuring messages are passed in this new landscape.

- **Cortical Remapping:**
 - Just as a business might repurpose an old space for new uses, the brain can assign new tasks to regions once dedicated to a lost sense, enabling them to process alternative inputs – this is the brain's way of renovating itself.

- **Role of Rehabilitation:**
 - Rehabilitation activities serve as the brain's training regimen, including tasks like sensory exercises and cognitive games that encourage neural growth and flexibility.
 - The repetitive nature of these exercises, much like practice in learning a musical instrument, solidifies the brain's adaptive responses, enhancing function over time.

This detailed exploration illustrates the brain's phenomenal adaptability – an internal resilience that parallels the spirit of a community rebuilding itself stronger and wiser. Each component of neuroplasticity plays a crucial role in this recovery, from the molecular support crew to the strategic remodeling of functions, reminding us of the astounding capability of our brains to heal and overcome.

Sensory perception is an everyday marvel where our senses collect information that the brain synthesizes into our experience of the world. This process begins with raw data – the sights, sounds, tastes, touches, and smells that surround us. Our brain, a masterful processor, interprets these signals, allowing us to navigate and interact with our environment. The significance of sensory perception extends beyond mere recognition of stimuli; it underpins our survival, communication, decision-making, and enjoyment of life. It influences our emotions and memories, and it plays a key role in all our social interactions. In essence, sensory perception is the foundation upon which we construct our understanding of reality, showcasing the brain's remarkable ability to transform sensory inputs into a coherent, meaningful, and personal portrait of the world we live in.

CONCLUSION

As we close the final pages of 'Neurology Made Easy', we reflect on a journey that has demystified the daunting intricacies of the human nervous system and brought to light the marvels of neurology. We've traversed from the fundamental structures of neurons to the complexities of neurological disorders, each concept explained with the aid of relatable analogies and vivid examples, making the sophisticated simple and the complicated clear.

Key themes have emerged throughout our exploration: the remarkable adaptability of the brain, the finely-tuned orchestra of neurological functions, and the crucial importance of neurological health in our overall well-being. We have learned the language of the brain, translated its silent messages, and understood its whispers and cries when in distress.

As we part ways with this guide, the book's impact lingers with a lasting impression of neurology's relevance in everyday life. The knowledge embraced here is more than academic; it's the recognition of our own biological narrative that unfolds within each of us. The intricacies of thought, the dance of neurotransmitters, and the resilience in recovery are but fragments of an elaborate tapestry that defines human experience.

May this book stand as a testament to the ever-evolving field of neurology and as a beacon for continued learning and curiosity. It is our hope that the layers of understanding built here inspire you to further unravel the mysteries of the nervous system and apply this knowledge with compassion and competence in both personal and professional spheres.

Remember, the study of neurology is not a final destination but an ongoing journey. Let the insights gained fuel questions for future discovery and remind us that within the complex wiring and chemical symphonies of our brains lies the profound narrative of what it means to be human.

ABOUT THE AUTHOR

Jon Adams brings a wealth of experience from over twenty years in the information technology industry, having worked with some of the world's leading tech giants. With a deep-seated passion for science, technology, and languages, Jon excels at demystifying complex subjects, making them accessible and engaging to a broad audience. His writings focus on breaking down intricate topics into everyday terms, helping readers not just learn but also apply this knowledge in their daily lives.

Currently, Jon is a proud member of Green Mountain Computing, which publishes his insightful books. Through his work, he aims to foster a deeper understanding and appreciation of technology and science, enriching readers' lives.

Jon@GreenMountainComputing.com

www.ingramcontent.com/pod-product-compliance
Lightning Source LLC
Chambersburg PA
CBHW071200240526
45470CB00017B/758